INTERMITTENT FASTING

The Complete Guide to Boost Your Metabolism, Gain Energy, Improve Weight Loss and Burn Fats for a healthy body.

By David Smith

Book1

book2

INTERMITTENT FASTING DIET

The complete Guide to healthy body healing through intermittent fasting and exact diet plan

Chapter 1. Introduction

There are a huge number of books composed on the point presenting distinctive eating less junk food plans for weight reduction clarifying the absolute most well-known sustenance approaches and considerably more. A considerable lot of these weight control plans propose removing certain macros, for example, cutting carbs or fats. Some of them recommend people should cut their everyday calorie admission, some propose an increment in active work.

There is without question a ton of going on, yet there is additionally one key factor which is absent in these eating less junk food plans. That factor is fasting, which is an experimentally demonstrated technique for bringing numerous medical advantages, assisting with weight reduction and significantly more.

Numerous individuals accept that fasting is tied in with starving, yet this isn't the situation. When fasting is done appropriately, it is one of those astoundingly powerful methodologies which can create stunning outcomes paying little mind to which eating less junk food plans you embrace.

1.1 What is Intermittent Fasting?

Intermittent fasting is a vague term for cycling between times of fasting and eating. There are a few kinds of intermittent fasting, yet they all offer one significant shared trait: Instead of zeroing in principally on what you eat, you focus harder on when you eat (albeit that doesn't mean the nature of your eating regimen isn't likewise significant).

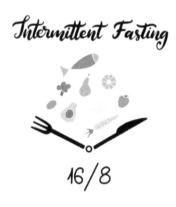

As indicated by Dr. Imprint Mattson, an analyst on intermittent fasting and teacher of neuroscience at Johns Hopkins University, the human body is intended to abandon nourishment for a few hours to a few days, however after the Industrial Revolution, food became available constantly. Subsequently, the human eating regimen changed altogether, and science hasn't got up to speed yet. Individuals are eating more food all the more regularly, and these additional calories (combined with stationary ways of life) have prompted ongoing medical problems like stoutness, type 2 diabetes, and coronary illness, which is the main source of death for ladies in the United States. At the point when you go for set timeframes without food, it permits your body to appropriately zero in on assimilation and exhaust your energy or glucose stores so your digestion is compelled to begin consuming your own muscle to fat ratio. Matt-child characterizes this cycle as "metabolic.

Intermittent fasting is a genuinely remedial methodology which can bring staggering outcomes in regards to weight reduction progress and by and large, both physical and emotional well-being in individuals who choose to accept it. Those people who are worn out on continually tallying their everyday calorie consumption, who are burnt out on fixating on the food sources they burn-through and who are basically worn out on disposing of their number one food sources from their eating routine, ought to clearly think about accepting the intermittent fasting way of life.

There are various advantages brought by an intermittent fasting way of life and one of them is that you don't need to surrender your number one food varieties helpful for arriving at your ideal weight and in compatibility of feeling incredible.

With intermittent fasting, people, truth be told, change their eating designs, they change when they eat, yet not what they eat. Consequently, there is no compelling reason to remove your number one food varieties, to stay away from delectable desserts and different food sources which are much of the time kept away from when following other well-known slimming down plans.

There is no more calorie tallying, no more fixating on your food sources and not any more battling with remaining progressing nicely. With intermittent fasting, you, truth be told, change your way of life adopting a straightforward steady strategy, you study eating fewer carbs propensities, their significance for your general wellbeing lastly, you figure out how to accept intermittent fasting for various medical advantages.

Regardless of your explanations behind being here, intermittent fasting is the best approach whether you need to normally get in shape, support your digestion, increment your energy or just feel incredible and sound each day.

To numerous individuals, intermittent fasting may seem like an exceptionally prohibitive methodology, as many accept that it is tied in with starving yourself, not eating routinely and other comparably false convictions. The book will break those false convictions. It will bring what you need to know on intermittent fasting, its medical advantages just as a basic, yet compelling bit by bit approach you can take helpful for benefiting from this slimming down way of life.

With the book, you will likewise find what the science is behind intermittent fasting backing up those various intermittent fasting benefits for your wellbeing. Furthermore, interestingly, you don't have to deny yourself of your best food sources for arriving at your wellbeing and counting calories objectives.

Intermittent fasting additionally furnishes stunning outcomes when joined with another mainstream, logically demonstrated weight reduction strategy known as the keto diet. At the point when you consolidate those intermittent fasting powers with the keto diet, you, truth be told, get the most forceful weight reduction.

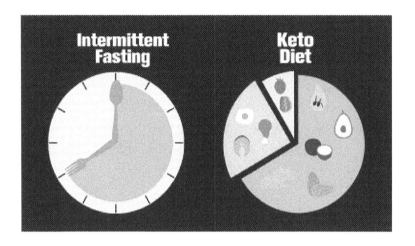

Both of these abstaining from excessive food intake plans are amazingly famous for various reasons. One of the primary reasons lies in the way that they bring various medical advantages as well as assisting with weight reduction progress. Before we get to those means you need to take toward fusing intermittent fasting into your way of life, we will talk about what intermittent fasting is, the thing that its advantages are and other significant snippets of data, so you can take a slow action towards this methodology.

It's critical that you make one stride at the time in assistance of creating your change as smooth as possible you have confidence that you have burned-through the perfect measures of supplements your body needs.

Truth be told, this is one of those objectives regardless of which consuming less calories plan you need to follow. You need to know every one of the significant realities before you really embrace your new abstaining from excessive food intake plan. As you do as such, you can make your eating fewer carbs progress totally smooth and you can make those progressions you will insight as could be expected. With this book, you will likewise study the significance of slimming down for both your physical and psychological well-being, you will realize what various sorts of consuming less calories plans are and their medical advantages.

Additionally, you will investigate how to benefit from intermittent fasting for boosting your weight reduction. The book likewise incorporates simple to follow, 30-day intermittent fasting difficulties which will assist you with accomplishing your ideal weight and lift your energy without battling.

As you investigate the book, you will, indeed, find a totally new, experimentally based way to deal with effortless weight reduction which can support your weight reduction venture as well as bring various other medical advantages your direction, which is something once in a while seen when following other eating fewer carbs plans.

You will investigate various ideas driving intermittent fasting; you will investigate various exercises on intermittent fasting which can bring about muscle acquire just as weight reduction.

With this book, you will likewise study distinctive intermittent fasting types which are presently overwhelming the whole wellness industry and substantially more which will help you draw nearer towards your weight and wellbeing objectives.

Exchanging." Keep as a primary concern that muscle versus fat is simply over the top food energy that has been put away; in the event that you keep on eating an overabundance, that abundance energy needs to discover some place to go, and muscle versus fat will keep on expanding. Then again, when you quick, your body goes to its own fat for a fuel source.

1.2 Fasting: A Historical Practice

As a custom, intermittent fasting is significantly more seasoned than the composed word. While utilizing it basically as a methods for weight reduction can be viewed as a moderately new wonder, it has a long history of utilization for things like heavenly correspondence, illness anticipation, improving fixation, diminishing the indications of maturing and then some. Fasting has been utilized by for all intents and purposes each religion and culture since the innovation of farming. Hippocrates, maybe the principal architect of current medication was rehearsing his exchange around 400 BC and quite possibly the most generally recommended medicines was of fasting routinely and drinking apple juice vinegar. He accepted (as it should be) that destroying takes fundamental assets through the stomach related cycle that the body could some way or another utilization for more beneficial cycles also. This thought came about in light of the fact that Hippocrates study the common tendency, everything being equal, to Ignore food while they are debilitated. Paracelsus, a contemporary of Hippocrates and the maker of the investigation of toxicology felt a similar way, venturing to such an extreme as to allude to the way toward fasting as the "doctor inside" in view of all the potential for great it can do in the human body. This inhabitant was afterward developed significantly more by in all honesty Benjamin Franklin who accepted that intermittent fasting was perhaps the most ideal approaches to fix a large group of normal illnesses. Strict works on; Fasting of some sort has consistently been seen by some as a profound practice which is likely why it is a significant inhabitant for religions all throughout the planet. Everybody from Buddha, to Muhammad, to Jesus Christ were completely known to lecture the advantages of fasting on a normal timetable. The Idea here is that the point of the training is to sanitize the physical or profound self, likely because of the increment in mental lucidity the interaction gives, with a scramble of its recuperating power tossed in just in case. Indeed, numerous Buddhists consistently eat in the first part of the day and afterward quick to the morning of the following day in request to feel considerably nearer to their confidence. Water diets that get longer and more as the expert ages are likewise very normal. With regards to Christianity, various groups quick for exacting time allotments for comparable reasons. The most limit illustration of this is maybe the Greek Orthodox Christians who quick for upwards of 200 days out of the year. Note that the Mediterranean Diet, which made it notable how solid individuals are around there, based quite a bit of it research in Crete which is generally Greek Orthodox. All things considered, It Is almost certain that intermittent fasting ought to be a characteristic piece of this eating routine also. In the biggest part of Christianity, Roman Catholicism, fasting Is conventional seen at a few central issues during that time and is for the most part rehearsed by eating one huge supper in the day just as two more modest dinners all at once that is near the main feast. This is most ordinarily seen on Ash Wednesday, which incorporates not eating any meat, and every one of the Fridays in the long stretch of Lent. While this isn't needed, it is mentioned by the individuals who are more established than 18 and under 59. This training as followed today is undeniably less exacting than it used to be preceding 1956. Other than nowadays, Roman Catholics are required to follow the occasion known by the name the Eucharistic Fast. This is the quick that should occur an hour before the time the expert realizes they will be taking mass. This time span used to stretch out between 12 am and the hour of Mass on Saturday however was abbreviated to where it doesn't give any genuine advantages but to get the body used to not eating. In the Bahai confidence, experts work on fasting every day for 12 hours during the period of March and they keep away from fluids notwithstanding food sources. Everybody in the confidence between the periods of IS and 70 is relied upon to take part on the off chance that they believe they can do it appropriately. Fasting is likewise consistently seen as a component of the Muslim confidence during Ramadan. This is a comparative light quick that even bars water. The prophet Muhammad was likewise referred to energize customary intermittent fasting also. Fasting is additionally a significant piece of the Hindu religion as it requests its supporters to notice a few distinct sorts from diets dependent on neighborhood custom and individual conviction. It is regular for some Hindus to quick certain days of every month. Moreover, the individual days of the week are additionally committed to fasting dependent on which god the expert is given to. The individuals who love Shiva commonly quick on Mondays, supporters of Vishnu keep an eye on quick on Thursdays and devotees of Ayyappa ordinarily quick on Saturdays. Fasting is additionally a typical piece of life in India where they consistently quick on explicit days. In numerous pieces of the country, they quick on Tuesdays in regard of the god called Lord Hanuman. This is a fluid just quick for the day however a few supporters will devour natural product also.

1.3 The Origin of Intermittent Fasting

Restorative fasting turned into a pattern during the 1800s as a method of forestalling or treating chronic weakness. Done under a specialist's oversight, this kind of fasting was embraced to get numerous conditions from hypertension migraines. Each quick was custom-made to the person's requirements. It very well may be only a day or as long as a quarter of a year.

In spite of the fact that fasting become undesirable as new prescriptions were created, it has as of late reappeared. In 2019, "intermittent fasting" was quite possibly the most ordinarily looked through terms. All in all, what would it be advisable for you to think about it?

1.4 Why is Intermittent Fasting Diet so popular?

Heftiness is turning into an expanding issue. Thus, it's no big surprise that such countless individuals are searching for a superior method to get more fit. Conventional weight control plans that confine calories frequently neglect to work for some individuals. It's hard to follow this sort of diet in the long haul. This frequently prompts yo-yo counting calories an interminable pattern of weight reduction and gain. Not exclusively does this frequently bring about emotional wellness issues, it can likewise prompt much more weight acquire generally.

It does not shock anyone, at that point, that numerous individuals have been looking for an eating regimen that can be kept up long haul. Intermittent fasting is one such eating routine. Even more a way of life change than an eating plan, it is unique in relation to ordinary eating regimens. Numerous supporters of intermittent fasting think that it's simple to follow for broadened periods. Far better, it assists them with getting more fit viably.

Nonetheless, this kind of eating plan additionally offers benefits past weight reduction. Numerous individuals accept that it can offer other wellbeing and health benefits as well. A portion of those advantages are even said to extend further some say it makes them more beneficial and centered. Thus, they can turn out to be more fruitful in the work environment. There have been late stories in the media of CEOs who guarantee their prosperity is all down to intermittent fasting.

However, the advantages don't stop there. There is some proof to show that intermittent fasting (or IF) helps health in alternate ways as well. It has been said to improve glucose levels and insusceptibility. It might support mind work, decline irritation and fix cells in the body as well.

In light of the entirety of this current, it's not difficult to perceive any reason why this method of eating is getting more well-known. Here, we'll investigate why intermittent fasting attempts to advance weight reduction. We'll look at the advantages of this way of life change and we'll tell you the best way to begin with this eating regimen convention.

1.5 How is Intermittent Fasting Different from Other Diet Plans?

Intermittent fasting (or IF for short) is a form of eating that occurs in lieu of a regular eating schedule. The focus in most eating plans is on the food you're eating. Weight watchers are restricted to a certain amount of calories or particular foods. Calorie counters will think about what they are and aren't allowed to eat as a result of this. Foods that are greasy or sweet are strictly forbidden. Vegetables, foods produced from the ground up, and low-sugar dinners are all getting a lot of attention. Many who practice these gobbling techniques often fantasies about sweets and bites. Though they may lose weight, they may struggle to stick to their diet in the long run.

Intermittent fasting is a one-of-a-kind practice. Rather than being a diet, it is a way of life. It involves eating plans that alternate between fasting and eating windows. It doesn't focus on the food you're consuming, unlike some other eating plans. When everything else is equal, it comes down to when you should feed. A few calorie counters enjoy the increased visibility this provides. They are free to consume the food sources that they enjoy. Many people even feel that it is more compatible with their lifestyles. In any case, there are certain possible pitfalls when it comes to using IF to lose weight.

1.6 The Most Popular Types of Intermittent Fasting Diet Plans

Intermittent fasting comes in a variety of forms. All has a distinct afterlife. Both adhere to the same standard of restricting food entry for a set period of time. Regardless, the amount of time between eating windows and the gap between them varies.

The 16:8 fast is perhaps the most well-known IF technique. This involves an 8-hour eating window followed by a 16-hour fast. Many people find this to be the most beneficial choice for them. They will easily incorporate skipping breakfast or supper into their daily routine.

Another famous IF choice is the 24-hour quick. This is now and then known as the Eat-Stop-Eat technique. It includes eating typically one day at that point staying away from nourishment for the accompanying 24 hours. The holes in the middle of diets could be just about as short as 24 hours or as long as 72 hours.

The 5:2 fasting technique is additionally mainstream. This includes eating typically for five days of the week. The other two back to back days, the weight watcher ought to limit their calorie utilization to around 500-600 calories.

A few IF weight watchers pick the 20:4 technique. This includes focusing all eating every day into a four-hour window. During the other 20 hours of the day, the weight watcher ought to eat no calories.

There are a few different sorts of fasting diet. A few group follow stretched out diets of up to 48 or 36 hours. Others quick for considerably more expanded periods. In case you're thinking about attempting IF, you'll need to pick the correct technique for you.

1.7 Why do People Prefer Intermittent Fasting Diet Plan?

In comparison to other methods of calorie restriction, IF allows calorie counters to consume just as much as they need. They can eat whatever sweet or greasy foods they want. They won't have to worry about calorie counting when they go out to eat. They don't have to eat foods they despise. They don't have to feel as if they're depriving themselves of their favorite items. It's not difficult to see why this is such a common decision.

That, however intermittent fasting offers a lot a bigger number of advantages than different sorts of diet. Indeed, it advances quick weight reduction. Nonetheless, it likewise assists calorie counters with feeling more engaged and be more beneficial. It assists them with feeling better and more enthusiastic. With the health benefits that this method of eating brings, it's no big surprise individuals lean toward it to normal weight control plans.

1.8 The Basics of Intermittent Fasting Diet Plan

The act of intermittent fasting has been around for innumerable hundreds of years and utilized for almost as a wide range of purposes. Notwithstanding, the explanation that a great many people have caught wind of the training these days is on account of its demonstrated capacity to help the individuals who practice it get thinner and keep it off in the long haul while simultaneously feeling more empowered than they have In years. The most awesome thing? Getting into the intermittent fasting way of life doesn't expect you to surrender the food varieties you adore or even eat less calories per supper. Indeed, the most usually utilized sort of intermittent fasting makes it feasible for the individuals who practice it to skip breakfast prior to eating two suppers later in the day. This kind of way of life change is ideal for the individuals who wind up experiencing difficulty staying with a stricter eating routine arrangement as it doesn't take a very remarkable change to begin seeing genuine outcomes, instead of being compelled to change everything at the same time. Indeed, this is the thing that settles on intermittent fasting an extraordinary decision for both the long and present moment as it is simple enough to begin with and stay with in the long haul and furthermore viable enough to produce ceaseless outcomes so the individuals who practice it are persuaded to keep up their great work.

The explanation that intermittent fasting is so fruitful is a direct result of the Incontrovertible truth that your body carries on distinctively when it is in a taken care of state rather than when it is in a fasting state. A took care of state is any timeframe when your body is at present retaining supplements from food while processing it. This state begins around five minutes after you have completed your supper and will stay for upwards of five hours relying upon the kind of feast it was and how troublesome It Is for your body to separate It into energy. While your body is in this state It Is continually delivering insulin, which makes it definitely more hard for the body to consume fat than it is when insulin creation isn't occurring?

The following old happens straightforwardly following processing before the abstained state has happened. It is known as the cushion period and it will then last anyplace somewhere in the range of eight and 12 hours dependent on what you last ate and individual body science. It is just during this flat, when your Insulin levels have gotten back to typical that your body will actually want to consume fat at top effectiveness. Because of the measure of time needed to arrive at a genuine fasting record, numerous individuals never feel its NH impacts as they seldom go eight hours without eating, considerably less 12. This doesn't mean making the progress is unimaginable, in any case, you should simply guarantee you exploit this normal state as a method of breaking the three squares a day propensity.

You might be hearing a great deal about intermittent fasting as of late, yet it's not new. Indeed, one of the most seasoned known logical examinations on intermittent fasting goes back 75 years! Furthermore, the idea overall returns considerably further to the times of chasing and assembling regardless of whether your progenitors weren't doing it deliberately. Intermittent fasting has stood the trial of time since it isn't simply one more eating regimen. It's an amazing eating system that has significant impacts when done effectively. While intermittent fasting can unquestionably assist you with shedding pounds, its medical advantages go far past that. It can likewise expand your energy, improve your fixation, lessen puffiness and aggravation, and help shield you and your mind from different persistent sicknesses. There's some disarray encompassing intermittent fasting, however. A few group believe it's simply an extravagant method of limiting calories, yet it's far beyond that. In this part, you'll get familiar with the essentials of intermittent fasting and why it's so incredible. You'll likewise find the distinction between intermittent fasting and calorie limitation and why you should kick low-calorie diets to the control until the end of time.

1.9 Intermittent Fasting Diet Plan Benefits

The fasting state is ideal with regards to shedding pounds and building muscle, however these are just two of the essential advantages of intermittent fasting. Perhaps the most startling advantages for some, individuals is the measure of time you will wind up saving when you abruptly don't need to stress over eating a whole feast, particularly in the event that you take the customary course and cut out breakfast, saving urgent time in what Is regularly the most feverish piece of the day for some individuals. Along comparable lines, you will likewise find that you have additional cash in your food spending plan as breakfast food sources are frequently the absolute priciest also. The distinction will probably be recognizable, regardless of whether you eat somewhat more all through the remainder of the day too. While the Idea of surrendering a whole feast each day may appear to be incomprehensible now, with training you will be shocked at how sensible it will turn into. It will absolutely be great also in light of the fact that, as well as guaranteeing there is additional time in your day and additional cash in your ledger, it can straightforwardly help you live a more extended, better life. Truth be told, examines show that when you invest additional time in the abstained express your body redirects that energy to its center endurance frameworks similarly it would when you are starving. While your body may see them as the equivalent for the time being, the truth is that the two states are incredibly unique which implies that the final product is that your body winds up revived by the interaction instead of being supported.

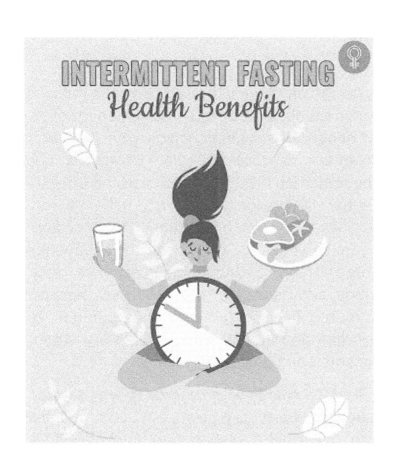

In particular, on the off chance that you invest a delayed time of energy in an abstained state you will enormously diminish your danger of stroke alongside your danger of a wide assortment of cardiovascular issues. It has additionally been demonstrated to decrease the impacts of chemotherapy in malignant growth patients too. Furthermore, these medical advantages don't require months or years to show up, they begin to arise when you start intermittent fasting and abatement your generally caloric admission by more than IS percent. Significantly more, benefits emerge as upgrades to regenerative organ and kidney work, circulatory strain, oxidative opposition and glucose resilience.

While all the 'Refined coarse with regards to why skirting a couple of suppers, every day prompts such emotional advantages isn't clear, what researchers have decided is that it is identified with the decrease of redundant pressure that the body encounters while fasting instead of eating three huge dinners daily. This is additionally why it improves the strength of the stomach related parcel just as that of numerous significant organs. It even gives the mitochondria in your body a lift, guaranteeing they use the energy accessible to them as productively as could really be expected. This, thus, has the additional gainful impact of diminishing the chances of oxidation harm happening anyplace in the framework.

The medical advantages to the body are eminent enough that both substitute days fasting, and numerous types of intermittent fasting are a medicinally affirmed method of diminishing one's danger of creating type 2 diabetes for the individuals who are now encountering the side effects of pre-diabetes. Presently, this advantage can absolutely be invalidated, which is the reason it is essential to not blame the way that you are fasting so as to feline everything and anything that you need, some restraint will in any case be required. This is the reason the most ideal decision is to not treat your time fasting as some extraordinary accomplishment, however to rather go about like it is only a normal piece of your daily practice. To see exactly how compelling intermittent fasting can be, consider a test that was performed on yeast cells that discovered when the yeast was denied of food its cells started to isolate all the more gradually accordingly. At the point when applied to your cells this means while you are fasting every one of your cells in a real sense lives longer than would some way or another be the case on account of this fake shortage. While the above rundown of medical advantages ought to be sufficient to in any event make the vast majority mull over Intermittent fasting prior to excusing it out and out, when they begin numerous individuals are amazed to And that something they appreciate most about the Intermittent fasting measure Is the way that it is a particularly basic yet gainful expansion to their day. It is so natural to use, truth be told, that in an investigation of those in excess of 30 pounds overweight, it was tracked down that more members had the option to adhere to an intermittent fasting plait than some other over a three-month timeframe. Additionally, while they were rehearsing intermittent fasting, this gathering of people saw a similar by and large measure of weight reduction as any other person. Maybe generally promising of all, in any case, Is that a year after the investigation had been finished, a greater amount of the individuals who had been intermittent fasting were as yet with it contrasted with the others and they had singularly lost the most weight by and large.

1.10 Getting started

With such countless advantages out there, you might be naturally restless to begin for yourself. To guarantee you can stay with the act of intermittent fasting as long as possible, nonetheless, there are a couple of rules you should remember. Buns more than you ear: While the Idea that you need to consume a bigger number of calories than you burn-through is a long way from progressive, it is particularly imperative to remember it while you are fasting irregularly as It can be far simpler to indulge post-quick than would some way or another be the situation, particularly when you are as yet becoming acclimated to the interaction.

In the event that you do slip, it very well may be not difficult to unnecessary the entirety of your diligent effort for the day with only a couple lost nibbles. There are 3,500 calories in a pound which implies that every week you need to consume at least 3,500 calories contrasted with what you devour in the event that you need to keep up your weight reduction consistently. While you may encounter a period where you are losing more than that as your body acclimates to the new way of eating, a consistent one pound seven days is the ideal sum as anything over that is unstainable In the long haul without at last putting your wellbeing in danger.

Continuously stay in charge: In request to utilize Intermittent fasting viably, it is essential that you have a suitable relationship with food directly from the beginning. On the off chance that you are the kind of individual who feels like certain food varieties, particularly their #1 food sources have a draw over them and your determination departs for good at the site of them then you may struggle beginning with intermittent fasting. Keep in mind, it is essential that you have the determination to go at least 12 hours without eating as any caloric admission will be sufficient to begin producing insulin and accordingly reset the clock. You should have the option to remove 500 calories from your eating routine, each day, to lose a pound seven days.

Suggestion: Download any wellness application to your cell phone it will help you gauge the number of calories you ought to burn-through consistently. While guaranteeing that you don't eat an excess of is a fundamental piece of the interaction, it is just a large portion of the fight as the other half is guaranteeing that you don't release yourself excessively long without eating. On the off chance that you expect to make intermittent fasting part of your life in the long-tens then it is imperative that you figure out how to add it to your life in a sound design as going excessively far one way or the other is simply going to prompt disappointment and possibly genuine wellbeing problems.

Stick with it: When it comes to utilizing Intermittent fasting consistently, It is Important to discover the variety that turns out best for you and afterward subside into a drawn out everyday practice rather than beginning and halting routinely. While you make certain to see a few outcomes immediately, it will require about a month for your body to completely acclimate to the interaction which implies you should be focused on the reason and patient just as nothing occurs without any forethought. While you make certain to get yourself incredibly eager, from the outset, after your body has realized when it can begin expecting calories you will find that your appetite pretty much gets back to business as usual. Besides, a month ought to be sufficient opportunity to begin seeing actual outcomes and indeed which ought to be sufficient to support your psychological grit considerably more. Then again, on the off chance that you quickly switch between strategies for intermittent fasting, or just use it for short blasts from time to time, at that point as opposed to upgrade your body's capacity to get more fit normally while additionally fabricating muscle, you will all things considered and it troublesome a lot of anything viably as your body will be In a consistent mess. All things considered, all weight reduction will stop as it attempts to cling to each and every calorie imaginable until it can sort out what on earth is going on. On the off chance that you really desire to see the kinds of results you are looking then the most ideal approach to guarantee this is the case is to discover one timetable of eating that works for you and afterward stay with it.

Converse with a medical care proficient: while the facts confirm that intermittent fasting assists individuals with getting thinner and fabricate muscle, notwithstanding a large group of different advantages, this doesn't mean it is naturally for everybody or that it doesn't book alongside some results too. First of all, when you first change to an intermittent fasting way of life you are probably going to encounter the runs, blockage or scenes of both for the initial fourteen days or so as your body acclimates to its new propensities. Moreover, it is imperative to be cautious in not allowing yourself to gorge adjust you have completed the process of fasting as this can prompt inner harm too. Notwithstanding how solid you intend to be; in any case, it is significant that you talk your arrangements over with either a dietitian or medical care proficient to guarantee you don't wind up unintentionally doing yourself more mischief than anything.

1.11 Women and Intermittent Fasting Diet Plans

While intermittent fasting is useful for the two people, men's bodies do take to the progress more effectively than ladies' bodies do. Accordingly, as a lady, on the off chance that you desire to make intermittent fasting a solid piece of your way of life then there are a couple of extra things you need to remember.

Numerous ladies who have attempted intermittent fasting recognize its various advantages. These incorporate decreased dangers of coronary illness, acquiring slender muscle, suggested glucose levels, diminished danger of persistent infections like disease and numerous others. Notwithstanding, alongside the great come hormonal changes inside their bodies that carry with them some different changes to a functioning way of life.

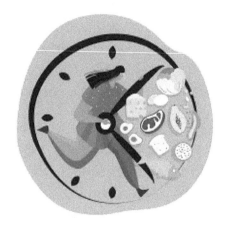

Nutrition deficiency: While embracing a intermittent fasting way of life, the main thing ladies need to remember is that the progress stage is likely going to interfere with the body's characteristic fruitfulness cycle. This is a protective component that is possibly disposed of when a satisfactory degree of sustenance Intake resumes. While fasting can influence your chemicals, intermittent fasting upholds legitimate hormonal equilibrium prompting a sound body and weight reduction the correct way once the body acclimates to the better approach for eating.

Additional challenges: While it isn't something that will influence everybody, a few ladies who routinely practice intermittent fasting do see issues like metabolic aggravations, beginning stage menopause, and missed periods. Likewise, on the off chance that you discover your body encountering delayed hormonal issues it could eventually prompt fair skin, balding, skin break out, diminished energy and the other, comparative issues. However long you don't take your fasting to the limit, at that point after the principal month or so you ought not to anticipate seeing any of these issues.

The explanation these hormonal Imbalances happen is that ladies are incredibly touchy to what exactly are known as starvation signals. All things considered, when a lady's body detects that it isn't accepting enough indispensable supplements it delivers a limit measure of the chemical's leptin and ghrelin to Increase the lady's longing to eat. All things considered, in the event that you find that you are totally eager when you arrive at the finish of your fasting stage then this could be the motivation behind why.

The explanation that ladies are quite a lot more helpless to this issue than men is to a great extent dependent on a protein called kisspeptin which is utilized by neurons to help in correspondence. It is additionally very touchy to ghrelin, leptin and insulin and present in far more noteworthy amounts in ladies than in men. At the point when the body produces exorbitant chemicals that quick you to eat, you are probably going to overlook them. Evidently, numerous ladies overlook these appetite signals, so the signs get much more Intense. The issue is that even these noisy signs are overlooked, and this may prompt gorging which can prompt the formation of a cycle that does little to guarantee your body gets the crucial supplements it needs while harming it in a larger number of ways than one. On the off chance that the negative propensities persevere for a really long time, it is conceivable that it can toss your chemicals messed up for all time.

Metabolism concerns: Your digestion Is Intimately attached to your wellbeing which implies that assuming you are encountering physiological or actual difficulties, your wellbeing could likewise be in danger. Fortunately, keeping a solid eating routine while working out, working out and fasting consistently would all be able to assist with settling these kinds of wellbeing challenges. Over the long haul, intermittent fasting has even appeared to assist offset with trip chemicals which implies you simply should know about the Issue and brave it while your body acclimates to your new propensities.

Protein concerns: Ladies will in general burn-through less protein contrasted with men. It follows then that fasting ladies devour even less protein. Less utilization of protein brings about less amino acids in the body. Amino acids are fundamental for the union of insulin-like development factor in the liver which initiates estrogen receptors. The development factor IGF-1 causes the uterine divider covering to thicken just as the movement of the conceptive cycle.

A delayed low protein admission can likewise influence your estrogen levels, which can likewise influence your metabolic capacity and the other way around. This can possibly influence your temperament, processing, insight, bone arrangement and that's only the tip of the iceberg. It can even influence the mind as estrogen is needed to invigorate the neurons liable for stopping the creation of the synthetics that direct hunger. Basically, any time your estrogen levels drop recognizably you are probably going to wind up feeling hungrier than would somehow or another be the situation.

As recently examined, ladies are normally more delicate to sensations of appetite than men are which is the reason numerous ladies find that fasting can be such a test. Fortunately, there is a variety of intermittent fasting that has been intended to locally available ladies all the more effectively into an intermittent fasting way of life. It is known as Crescendo Fasting and to follow it, you should simply begin by fasting three days every week on nonconsecutive days. You will find that you actually see a large number of the general advantages of intermittent fasting, without exposing yourself to the potential for hormonal awkwardness. This methodology is far gentler on the body during the progress time frame and it can assist you with changing fasting as fast as could really be expected. Assuming you still and that you are having issues, you can begin your day with around 250 calories prior to continuing to proceed with your quick as should be expected.

Advantages: The advantages of this style of intermittent fasting are for the most part In accordance with what the more thorough variants gloat and include:

• You acquire energy

• Improving provocative markers

• Losing weight and muscle versus fat

• No hormonal difficulties

Crescendo fasting Rules:

Above all, it is important that you do not fast for more than three days a week during the main month and never for more than 24 hours at a time. During these fasting times, you will need to fast for somewhere between 12 and 16 hours; it is important that you do not fast for more than 16 hours at a time if at all possible. When you do fast, you'll always need to work out, so do something light or wait until after you've broken your quick to start. While you are fasting, you are still allowed to drink water. As long as you don't add something calorie-dense to your espresso or tea, you're good to go. If you think you'll be close to the 16-hour mark, you may want to add some coconut oil and grass-fed margarine to your espresso. This approach to fasting informs your body that it is the perfect time for your cells to eat fat in order to obtain energy and clean up their act. For women, crescendo fasting has a distinct benefit.

It will also contribute to your wealth and appeal. After two or three weeks, you will notice the benefits that come with it.

- Radiant skin

- Healthy moxie

- Shiny hair

- A lively attitude

- Appropriate body weight

On the off chance that you are beyond 90 a few years old, in excess of a couple of pounds overweight, at that point you should consider adding grass-took care of collagen to your espresso on your fasting days all things being equal. Collagen can reset your leptin levels which will help battle hunger. During fasting days it is critical to keep both your fructose and sugars levels to a base as this will assist with advancing leptin levels in the body.

Chapter 2: The Importance of Nutrition

You're day by day abstaining from excessive food intake decisions unquestionably have a huge effect with regards to your actual wellbeing as well as to your emotional wellness state. Individuals are typically mindful of the way that having great nourishment and participating in actual work can help them keep up that ideal weight, yet in addition keep up their general wellbeing.

All things considered, truly the significance and advantages of having great nourishment and following a solid counting calories plan go a long ways past keeping up that ideal weight. Truly the food varieties you eat bring numerous other medical advantages, for example, diminishing the danger of building up certain sicknesses like diabetes, stroke, coronary illness, osteoporosis, a few malignant growths and others.

The food varieties you eat likewise can assist with the decrease of hypertension, they can help you lower elevated cholesterol levels, assist you with improving your general prosperity, improve your capacity to ward off various types of sicknesses, improve your capacity to recuperate from wounds and illness just as help you increment your energy levels.

2.1 What is Nutrition?

Nourishment likewise is known as sustenance. Sustenance is viewed to as the stockpile of various materials or food sources which are needed by the body and the body's cells instead of creating and stay alive.

In human medication and science, nourishment is viewed as the training or study of using and burning-through food varieties. Likewise, in clinical focuses and medical clinics, nourishment additionally may allude to the specific patients' food prerequisites including distinctive healthful arrangements which are conveyed by means of intra gastric cylinders or through intravenous.

In all actuality the human body requires a few significant nourishment types for improvement, development and remaining alive. There are additionally some pivotal supplements which don't furnish the body with energy, yet they are still critical like fiber and water, notwithstanding macronutrients for remaining alive.

With regards to macronutrients, they are critical, as without devouring them, it is difficult to work. Notwithstanding macronutrients the body needs, we likewise need different arrangements, for example, minerals and nutrients which are additionally urgent natural mixtures.

As hereditary qualities advance, organic chemistry and sub-atomic science, just as sustenance definitely have gotten an ever increasing number of zeroed in on various metabolic pathways digestion all in all. Nourishment clarifies diverse biochemical strides, through which various arrangements or substances inside the body are being changed, utilized as fuel sources.

Nourishment as a science is likewise committed to clarifying how unique medical problems and distinctive ailments can be decreased or even forestalled with great sustenance and sound consuming less calories draws near. Along these lines, nourishment likewise includes assessments on how unique ailments and infections can be brought about by certain dietary factors like food sensitivities, unhealthiness brought about by a horrible eating routine just as various food prejudices.

Appropriately, nourishment is viewed as the admission of various food varieties corresponding to the human body's dietary requirements. Hence, great sustenance is viewed as a sound and sufficient just as a reasonable eating fewer carbs plan which when joined with a standard exercise approach brings about great wellbeing.

Then again, helpless abstaining from excessive food intake decisions can prompt expanded defenselessness to various types of infections, diminished invulnerability, and hindered both mental and actual advancement just as extraordinarily decreased efficiency.

It can likewise be said that nourishment is the cycle by which people devoured and used diverse food substances in any case; those fundamental supplements which incorporate fat, protein, carbs, nutrients, electrolytes and minerals.

Around the vast majority of our everyday energy use comes from carbs and fats while around fifteen percent of our day by day energy use comes from burned-through proteins.

In people, nourishment is accomplished through the critical cycle of burning-through food varieties. With regards to the necessary measures of those fundamental supplements, these vary starting with one individual then onto the next relying upon their age, their condition of the body like their active work, meds taken and other clinical components.

2.2 What is Good Nutrition?

As recently referenced, great nourishment is unquestionably the main factor with regards to keeping up both great physical and psychological wellness states.

Indeed, eating an even eating routine is an urgent piece of having great wellbeing for each individual regardless of their age, ailments and different variables which vary starting with one individual then onto the next.

Sustenance as the examination or the study of various supplements contained in food varieties we burn-through, likewise shows us how the body really utilizes these various supplements just as shows us the connection between infection, wellbeing, and our consuming less calories decisions.

In the event that your nourishment is acceptable, it implies that you burn-through every one of those fundamental supplements your body needs for working at its best levels.

In the event that your consuming less calories decisions are acceptable, you shield yourself from different sorts of ailments and infections like coronary illness, heftiness, stroke, malignancy, diabetes, and numerous others.

Sadly, today numerous individuals rotate their slimming down decisions around immersed fats, sugars, or trans fats just as more sodium-stuffed vegetables and organic products. With these helpless counting calories decisions, the body's wellbeing may decay as it considers what we devour each day.

Settling on helpless slimming down decisions, indeed, decreases by and large prosperity, causes various issues with weight, for example, weight gain or weight reduction, harms the safe framework, makes us drained and fomented.

Helpless counting calories decisions additionally accelerate those maturing impacts, increment the dangers of building up certain illnesses, and contrarily influences the state of mind, diminishes both concentration and efficiency and numerous other amazingly adverse consequences.

As should be obvious, those food decisions you make each day altogether influence your general wellbeing, influencing how you will feel today, how you will tomorrow and how you will feel later on. Therefore, having a decent, even eating regimen is quite possibly the most vital advances prompting having a better way of life.

Actually an even eating regimen, when joined with a normal active work of any sort, can help you draw nearer towards your ideal weight, assist you with keeping up your ideal load just as decrease your dangers of creating diverse ailments.

2.3 Calculating your Body Mass Index

As recently expressed in the book, nourishment is critical for both turn of events and development just as for generally prosperity and by and large wellbeing.

Eating an even eating routine to just contributes emphatically to your physical and psychological wellness state, yet in addition adds to forestalling sicknesses prompting gigantic enhancements in your day to day existence quality and your life expectancy. With regards to your wholesome status, it is viewed as your general condition of wellbeing dictated by the food varieties you eat.

There are a few unique ways with regards to evaluating your generally speaking dietary situations with as your everyday food admission, your biochemical estimations, and your actual body estimations or your anthropometric estimations.

One of those vital markers of your overall nourishing status is your BMI or your weight list. Your BMI considers your tallness and your weight just as corresponds with the aggregate sum of fat you have, which is for this situation communicated as a specific level of your body weight.

It ought to be noticed that the genuine connection communicated in BMI details rely upon age following the most noteworthy relationship was found in people of ages between 26 and 55 years while the least relationship is found in the older populace.

To compute your BMI status or your weight record, you need to take your weight communicated in kilograms and separation it by your stature communicated in meters squared. That number you get communicates your weight list. It ought to be noticed that those higher qualities show more noteworthy fat stores entire those lower number demonstrate deficient stores of fat.

When you have your weight list decided, it tends to be exceptionally useful filling in as your own analytic device whether you are underweight or overweight.

On the off chance that your weight list number if somewhere in the range of 25 and 29, you are overweight while a weight record number which is over 3o arranges as fat.

You should press towards having a solid weight record which is somewhere in the range of 18.5 and 24.9. As well as deciding your general nourishment status, weight record likewise computes the measure of fat contained in the body which is particularly significant for competitors, ladies who are pregnant and jocks.

Weight list generally speaking overestimates the fat sum in the body for these gatherings while it belittles the fat contained in the body in old individuals just as in people who battle with some sort of actual incapacity, who have issues with their muscles or who can't walk.

It ought to be noticed that that in spite of these advantages weight list isn't the absolute best proportion of wellbeing and weight hazard as there is likewise an abdomen condition which should be considered with regards to foreseeing wellbeing chances.

In addition, that wellbeing weight record scope of 20 to 25 is just appropriate for grown-ups and not for kids. Truth be told, for grown-up individuals who have quit creating and growing, an increment in their weight list is most much of the time brought about by a critical expansion in their muscle to fat ratio.

Then again, kids who are as yet during the time spent developing and creating, their fat sum in the body changes after some time which likewise causes changes in their weight record.

Consequently, weight list diminishes during those preschool years while it will in general increment as we enter adulthood. Consequently, a weight list for youths and kids should be looked at considering their age just as their sexual orientation outlines.

2.4 Calculating your Waist Circumference

As referenced in the past part of the book, another extraordinary apparatus you can use for deciding your wellbeing chances, as well as utilizing your weight list, is your abdomen perimeter.

Truth be told, your midsection outline is a far superior wellbeing hazard indicator than simply weight list. Truly having a potbelly or having fat around your midsection regardless of your real size brings more wellbeing chances, particularly for those stoutness related ailments.

Truth be told, fat which is predominately arranged around the midsection is more perilous than fat which is arranged around the rump and hips. There are various investigations directed on the subject which recommend that the appropriation of those fat sources is related with various wellbeing dangers, for example, having more elevated cholesterol levels, creating heart illnesses or diabetes.

Lesser wellbeing chances are identified with having no potbelly or being thin around here while moderate danger is identified with being overweight, however having no potbelly. The more serious danger from moderate to high danger is identified with being thin, however having a potbelly and high danger is identified with being overweight and having a potbelly.

Since abdomen outline is identified with a wide range of wellbeing chances, it is a smart thought that you measure your midsection. For men, having at least 94 centimeters in the midsection shows an expanded danger while having at least 102 in centimeters around the midriff demonstrates a generously expanded wellbeing hazard.

The numbers are somewhat less for ladies. Having at least eight centimeters around the midsection for ladies shows a marginally expanded danger while having 88 centimeters around the abdomen demonstrates a considerably expanded danger.

It ought to be noticed that accepting standard actual work, keeping away from undesirable propensities, for example, smoking and burning-through more unsaturated fats rather soaked fats can diminish the danger of creating issues related with stomach weight.

2.5 Why is Nutrition Important?

The effect of the eating fewer carbs decisions you make each day add to various spaces of your general wellbeing influencing both your physical and psychological wellness state. Truth be told, there have been various examinations directed on the point which propose that undesirable eating less junk food decisions have altogether added to the huge heftiness scourge in the US.

A similar report likewise recommended that around 33% of grown-ups in the United States, which is in excess of about a third of grown-up residents, are battling with corpulence. The numbers are not extraordinary for kids and young people either, as a similar report has proposed that in excess of seventeen millions youths and offspring of ages two to nineteen are likewise large.

Besides, even those people who have a sound weight additionally can battle with various ailments having some significant dangers which can cause diseases and sometimes even passing. These incorporate creating type 2 diabetes, having hypertension or hypertension, battling with osteoporosis or in any event, building up certain sorts of malignant growth.

Subsequently, it is critical that you center around changing your unfortunate eating designs by settling on keen decisions rotating around your eating regimen, you, truth be told, can shield yourself from various medical problems.

There are some other danger factors identified with helpless counting calories decisions like the advancement of certain sorts of persistent infection, which are lamentably progressively seen in grown-ups as well as in kids and youths of more youthful ages.

Truly the dietary propensities we have set up in our adolescence frequently keep during our adulthood years. Therefore, it is critical that guardians give time to showing their kids great nourishment, and how to eat quality food varieties. Truth be told, that connection between having great nourishment and having great weight altogether lessens the danger of building up those sorts of constant sicknesses; it is excessively significant for us to disregard it.

Therefore, it is critical to you find certain ways to accept a better, even eating routine which will help you fuel your body with the entirety of the significant supplements your body needs for working at its best, remaining solid, dynamic and sound.

Furthermore, very much like with expanding your actual work and accepting other sound propensities, rolling out these little improvements in your counting calories example can lead you far. At the point when you embrace an even eating regimen loaded with entire grains, vegetables, and organic products, you fulfill your craving levels as well as you simultaneously feed your general body.

Despite the fact that it is totally fine to enjoy some less quality food sources occasionally, it is critical that you're eating routine incorporates those fundamental supplements your body needs for endeavoring.

2.6 Benefits of Good Nutrition

In this part of the book, we will talk about additional a portion of the fundamental advantages of settling on great dietary decisions. One of them is that acceptable sustenance can essentially improve your general prosperity. Very much like eating less nutritious food sources diminishes both your psychological and actual wellbeing, people who devour food sources wealthy in supplements are less inclined to report having issues with their psychological and actual wellbeing.

Since eating permits us to be more dynamic as we have more energy, around 66% of people who routinely burn-through new vegetables and new natural products report no serious issues with their general wellbeing state. This is simple contrasted with those people who have some sort of emotional well-being problem who by and large have a terrible eating routine, and eat less nutritious food varieties.

In compatibility of securing your general prosperity and your general wellbeing state, your food decisions ought to incorporate those fundamental supplements which will be talked about in the following segment of the book.

Settling on the correct slimming down decisions additionally forestalls the advancement of different sicknesses. Indeed, having great nourishment and even dietary patterns can decrease your danger of building up certain sorts of coronary illness, type 2 diabetes or having hypertension and raised cholesterol levels.

Normally, keeping up great nourishment additionally assists you with remaining in the correct shape, assisting you with the upkeep of your ideal weight. Eating normal food sources rather than handled food sources decidedly impacts your weight just as your general wellbeing state.

In actuality, being overweight builds your dangers for creating ongoing conditions, for example, type 2 diabetes, which when left untreated, can restrict your versatility while harming your joints. Thus, toward remaining fit as a fiddle, you're eating routine ought to incorporate a lot of entire grains, vegetables, products of the soil food sources wealthy in fundamental supplements.

Truth be told, keeping an even eating regimen notwithstanding standard actual work is the best way to get thinner and keep up it over the long haul. There is no supernatural pill or enchanted beverage which may assist people with losing those extra pounds. There are just acceptable sustenance and an expansion in actual work as the regular method of shedding pounds.

Individuals regularly battle with famous eating less junk food plans as they for the most part confine their #1 food varieties. This can work in the short run as people for the most part embrace their old eating fewer carbs propensities for quite a while. Toward staying away from this issue, the best thought is to rethink those old plans, add a few tones with those new veggies, and mix it up.

It is likewise critical to treat yourself for certain less good food sources now and again as everything is about balance. It isn't tied in with confining yourself from those food sources you appreciate, however it is tied in with adding some more to them. Truth be told, adding new veggies and organic products can have an immense effect assisting you with controlling your cholesterol levels, and your circulatory strain just as your weight.

This is actually where intermittent fasting goes to the game. Rather than fixating on your day by day calorie admission, rather than eating food varieties that you abhor, you figure out how to change your present consuming less calories examples and spotlight on when you eat rather than what you eat. Today it is incredibly costly to be undesirable. In all actuality individuals battling with consuming less calories decisions are bound to build up some sort of ailments because of their helpless eating fewer carbs decisions and being debilitated accompanies costs.

Thus, there is nothing unexpected in the way that in excess of over two thirds of the medical care and clinical consideration dollars in the United States are spent on treating preventable illnesses identified with consuming less calories decisions. You likely have encountered eating a lot of food varieties and out of nowhere getting a charge out of an explosion of energy just to feel totally depleted in an exceptionally brief timeframe later.

This happens in light of the fact that the body responds upon those food sources containing countless refined sugars. In expanding energy levels which will last subsequent to devouring food varieties, you need to stay away from unfortunate food sources and spotlight on burning-through food varieties which are loaded with fundamental supplements your body will use as its fuel.

As you embrace great eating less junk food decisions, you can at long last build your energy levels which will last for the duration of the day, not for only a few hours and in particular, you won't encounter those standard fail spectacularly impacts.

Besides, you will actually want to zero in additional on what's going on around you, which isn't the situation when you feel depleted and tired. As you most likely are aware, the body gets energy from those food varieties we ingest just as from fluids we devour.

The fundamental supplements the body utilizes as its energy powers are protein, fats, and carbs. Those carbs like entire grains, boring vegetables, and bread are the best fuel sources since they are processed much slowly. Additionally, water is likewise one of those fundamental components vital for supplement transportation.

Lick of water or parchedness can prompt absence of energy, so as much it is critical to burn-through those fundamental supplements, it is additionally essential to keep your body hydrated. Furthermore, an iron inadequacy can likewise cause low energy levels and peevishness just as weariness. Hence, you're eating regimen ought to likewise remember food varieties rich for iron; verdant veggies like spinach, peas, and poultry just as fish.

In compatibility of acquiring the most from these food sources, the best thought is to build your nutrient C admission simultaneously. Consider adding a greater amount of those nutrient C-rich food sources like verdant greens, broccoli, tomatoes, kiwi and peppers.

Great sustenance likewise assists with keeping your invulnerable framework working at its best. As you probably are aware, our insusceptible framework helps us battling ailments and sicknesses, and yet, having helpless sustenance implies your resistant framework is harmed, so it can't work as expected.

For keeping up your resistant framework, your body requires a specific admission of those fundamental supplements just as legitimate minerals and nutrients. Henceforth, eating an even eating routine loaded with those supplements can help you support your resistant framework.

Great nourishment additionally can assist with your skin wellbeing just as help you postpone maturing impacts. Eating an even eating routine not just influences your energy levels, your safe framework, and your weight yet in addition assumes a pivotal part with regards to your skin wellbeing.

As per the most recent examinations directed on the theme, food sources which are plentiful in nutrient E and C, wealthy in cell reinforcements and lycopene help additionally help shield your skin from sun harm. Food varieties like nuts, avocados, berries, tomatoes, and fish all come loaded with fundamental minerals and supplements which are astounding for the skin.

For example, tomatoes are loaded with nutrient C that helps in the structure of collagen that improves the skin, firmer and smoother which postpones maturing impacts. What's more, berries are additionally extraordinary for the skin as they are loaded with nutrients and cell reinforcements which advance skin recovery keeping your skin smooth, firm and new.

As referenced already, accepting a decent eating regimen likewise implies you decrease your danger of building up certain sorts of persistent infections, for example, hypertension, type a diabetes and other.

These danger factors are fundamentally expanded in people who are overweight or who eat horribly. In feet, among grown-up people between ages reason for visual deficiency, kidney disappointment, and amazingly removal.

Burning-through good food sources can decidedly influence your mind-set just as your generally speaking emotional well-being state. Consuming less calories plans which are limited in starches admission normally increment those pressure sentiments while eating less junk food plans which advance carbs accompany considerably more inspiring impacts influencing mind-set.

Likewise, eating less junk food plans which are wealthy in proteins, low in fat and moderate in carbs additionally have significantly constructive outcomes on emotional well-being and state of mind since they give the body sufficient omega 3-unsaturated fats and iron supplies.

Similarly as the food varieties we burn-through influence our disposition, the state of mind can likewise influence our dietary decisions. At the point when we are tragic, we are bound to settle on undesirable dietary decisions while individuals who are more joyful are bound to pick better food sources.

Great nourishment, notwithstanding these medical advantages, additionally assists us with expanding our efficiency and core interest. Truly the food sources we devour hugely affect the manner in which we feel and think. For example, when your body is coming up short on glucose, you are less inclined to think and center, as the cerebrum isn't accepting sufficient energy.

Counting calories plans which are extremely high in cholesterol and fat, indeed, can seriously harm the cerebrum by building plaque sources inside mind vessels which further harm the tissues of the cerebrum.

Thus, you ought to keep away from food varieties loaded with outrageous measures of fat and spotlight on eating more veggies and organic products which will help you remain on track and beneficial for the duration of the day.

Another stunning medical advantage of good sustenance is that it can stretch your life. As you most likely are aware, the body needs food varieties and supplements for developing, creating and enduring. Then again, the way toward separating food supplements, the way toward processing them, can make an enormous pressure the body.

Consequently, indulging makes more pressure the body which can cause a more limited life expectancy. As indicated by the most recent investigation directed on the theme, around eighteen percent of passing among American residents are added to stoutness.

In this way, being corpulent can prompt a huge decrease in by and large future in the United States as well as when all is said in done. The best thought is to accept dietary decisions which are loaded with fundamental supplements and stay away from handled food sources which cause more pressure to the body.

As you can see from this section, your dietary decisions influence your stomach as well as influence each organ in the body including your skin, mind, your heart, resistant framework and all the other things. Consequently, great sustenance can bring various medical advantages to ensuring and aiding you on a wide range of levels while expanding the general nature of your life.

Conclusion

Intermittent fasting, when embraced for wellbeing reasons in patients with diabetes mellitus, the two kinds 1 and 2, has been appeared in a couple of little human examinations to prompt weight reduction and diminish insulin necessities. While these discoveries are energizing and have caught the creative mind of numerous individuals, an astute way to deal with executing fasting regimens and utilizing them in the long haul among this particular populace is required. A significant part of the promotion encompassing fasting emerges from creature examines, which just propose what human exploration ought to be directed; execution of human intercessions ought not to be founded on creature research.

Long haul advantages of fasting, including cardiovascular danger decrease, stay to be completely considered and clarified, particularly in people. Clinicians should temper the eagerness for fasting with the truth that the advantages and dangers in people remain to a great extent neglected and the advantages may require a long time to years to show up or be completely figured it out. Great proof from epidemiologic investigations, pilot interventional preliminaries, and a couple of randomized preliminaries recommends that the advantages of fasting exceed the likely damages in the normal person. Individuals with diabetes, be that as it may, are not the normal individual, and their own necessities require more cautious thought toward the start of and during the utilization of a fasting routine. With legitimate drug change and observing of blood glucose levels however, intermittent fasting can be supported and securely executed among individuals with diabetes.

INTERMITTENT FASTING

The Easy and Sustainable Way to a Healthy Life Style Step-by-step

presentation of the information is without a contract or any guarantee assurance.The trademarks used are without any consent, and the publication of the trademark is without permission or backing by the trademark owner. All trademarks and brands within this book are for clarifying purposes only and are owned by the owners themselves s, not affiliated with this document.

Corpulence stays a significant general wellbeing concern and intermittent fasting is a mainstream procedure for weight reduction, which may introduce autonomous medical advantages. Nonetheless, the quantity of diet books exhorting how fasting can be fused into our day by day lives is a few significant degrees more noteworthy than the quantity of preliminaries looking at whether fasting ought to be supported by any means. This survey will consider the condition of current arrangement with respect to different types of intermittent fasting (for example 5:2, time-limited taking care of and substitute day fasting). The adequacy of these transiently characterized approaches shows up extensively comparable to that of standard day by day energy limitation, albeit a considerable lot of these models of intermittent fasting don't include took care of abstained cycles each and every other 24 hours rest wake cycle and additionally license some restricted energy consumption outside of endorsed taking care of times. In like manner, the intercession time frame along these lines may not consistently substitute, may not traverse all or even the vast majority of some random day, and may not include supreme fasting. This is significant in light of the fact that possibly favorable physiological systems may possibly be started if a post-absorptive state is supported by continuous fasting for a more drawn out length than applied in numerous preliminaries. In fact, promising consequences for fat mass and insulin affectability have been accounted for when fasting span is regularly stretched out past sixteen continuous hours. Further advancement will require such models to be tried with suitable controls to seclude whether any conceivable wellbeing impacts of intermittent fasting are principally owing to routinely extended post-absorptive periods, or essentially to the net negative energy balance by implication inspired by any type of dietary limitation.

Weight is a pervasive wellbeing worry all through the world, which emerges because of persistent positive energy balance. Any energy excess is put away basically as TAG inside adipocytes, consequently prompting fat tissue development prevalently because of adipocyte hypertrophy. Whenever supported after some time, this hypertrophic extension can prompt adipocyte brokenness, hyperglycemia, hyperlipidemia, ectopic lipid affidavit, constant poor quality foundational aggravation and insulin opposition, subsequently encouraging comorbidities, for example, type 2 diabetes and CVD. To cure this metabolic brokenness, mediations frequently try to change the hidden energy awkwardness by diminishing energy admission or potentially expanding use, which can improve wellbeing results. Nonetheless, these upgrades are hampered by compensatory changes in hunger and energy use, just as helpless adherence, bringing about poor long haul achievement rates.

Methodologies that endeavor supplement timing as a methods for accomplishing weight reduction or potentially improving metabolic wellbeing have been the subject of extensive public interest as of late. Intermittent fasting is an umbrella term that might be utilized to portray these methodologies, which include a total or incomplete limitation of energy inside characterized fleeting windows on a repetitive premise. Up to this point, the helpful capability of intermittent fasting has been generally eclipsed by direct control of the vital parts of the energy balance condition. Notwithstanding, progresses in the comprehension of circadian rhythms propose that this could be an especially viable methodology for handling corpulence and the going with brokenness, as well as seemingly being more adequate practically speaking than regular other options. To investigate this thought, this survey will consider the writing on dinner timing and intermittent fasting as it identifies with metabolic wellbeing.

1.1 Meal timing

In Western societies, burning-through at least three suppers every day is by and large acknowledged as a cultural standard. Notwithstanding, this normally brings about an anabolic state prevailing every day. The postprandial metabolic reaction to a blended macronutrient supper in metabolically sound members is described by a top in glycaemia inside the main hour followed by a consistent re-visitation of abstained glycaemia over the resulting 2 hours. This is resembled by a going with top in insulin discharge inside the principal hour followed by a lessening throughout the following 4 hours. Alternately, plasma TAG focuses rise consistently to a top after 3–5 h and for the most part stay 50 % higher than pattern even following 6 hours. At the point when a resulting supper is ingested roughly 5 hours after the first (as is regular in Western eating regimens), glucose tops at a comparative time subsequent to taking care of, but a lessened outright pinnacle. Nonetheless, glucose at that point takes marginally more to get back to standard as the day advances, an example that is to a great extent reflected by insulin focuses. Plasma TAG then again doesn't top until not long after the subsequent dinner is ingested; it at that point falls quickly due to the insulinaemic reaction to the subsequent supper, prior to cresting again around 5 hours after the subsequent feast.

INTERMITTENT
FASTING

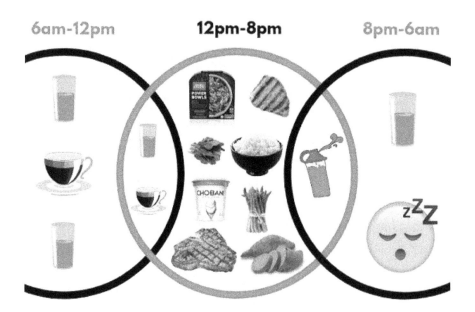

6am-12pm   **12pm-8pm**   8pm-6am

These reactions propose that, even with only two suppers every day, plasma TAG is raised ceaselessly for 12 hours, with this example at that point proliferated when further stretched out to incorporate a third dinner. This is very much exhibited by scientist, who analyzed the 24 hours flowing profiles of glucose, TAG and insulin because of three progressive dinners at 10.00, 15.00 and 20.00 hours. Inside this model, TAG stayed raised until 02.00 hours, alongside insulin and glucose fixations. Also, it is showed that TAG extraction by fat tissue because of three dinners every day is raised for more than 16 hours. The net impact of this is that most of every 24 h day is spent in a postprandial and lipogenic state, which is helpful for fat gradual addition. Likewise, this gives less freedoms to net lipolysis and the prevalence of lipid-inferred substrates in energy digestion, consequently preferring positive fat equilibrium.

Eventually, this outcomes in a situation wherein those clinging to customary dietary dinner timing designs are endeavoring to accomplish energy balance utilizing a taking care of timetable that is intrinsically one-sided towards fat accumulation. Customary eating routine and exercise mediations plan to lessen the abundance of postprandial journeys to give more freedoms to the freedom and usage of endogenous lipid supplies. Nonetheless, the unevenness between the everyday fasting window and the day by day taking care of window remains to a great extent unperturbed. Nearly, the oversight of dinners is normally required by intermittent fasting and disposes of a subset of these postprandial outings, accordingly giving more noteworthy balance among fasting and taking care of chances and a superior stage for accomplishing energy balance.

Further to this, the normal augmentation of fasting periods has been related with metabolic advantages which are free of net energy balance, establishing an auxiliary restorative measurement to these methodologies. In particular, it is contend that the consumption of hepatic glycogen holds and the following change towards digestion of endogenous, lipid-inferred substrates (for example glycerol, ketone bodies) brief a progression of versatile cycles helpful for improved wellbeing results, remembering upgrades for body piece and insulin affectability. Taking into account that this change doesn't occur in many cases until the continuous fasting length continues past 12–14 hours, these versatile cycles are not frequently conjured by the traditional feast designs portrayed before.

In light of the before referenced thinking, it is possible that intermittent fasting may comprise a solid system for handling stoutness and the metabolic issues related with overabundance adiposity. Until this point, nonetheless, contemplates investigating these features of intermittent fasting are scant and conflicting.

Maybe the most broadly investigated measurement of supplement timing inside the setting of weight in human subjects is eating recurrence. Early work sent a cross-sectional way to deal with investigate the connection between admission recurrence and metabolic wellbeing. Curiously, in a partner of 440 men, higher eating recurrence extensively compared to a better profile of BMI, cholesterol focuses and fasting glucose. In spite of this, utilizing information from the public wellbeing and nourishment assessment overview, seen that those eating on multiple events every day were roughly 50 % bound to be overweight or corpulent by BMI comparative with those eating on under three events day by day. Such errors are a steady subject all through these cross-sectional examinations; a new orderly survey dissected information from 31 such investigations containing an aggregate example of more than 130 000 members. Of these 31 examinations, fourteen set up a backwards affiliation, ten showed no affiliation and seven uncovered a positive affiliation, which the creators attribute to the range of approaches utilized.

After moving to forthcoming approaches, the example seems, by all accounts, to be generally something very similar; two late methodical surveys reason that most of studies uncover no relationship between eating recurrence and resulting heftiness. The survey makes an especially solid case, given that these creators just remembered human investigations for which food was given or admission observed in a research facility setting. In any case, of the examinations canvassed in these surveys, most assessed the effect of expanded supper recurrence on metabolic wellbeing, wherein three dinners every day is utilized as the reference for lower recurrence. Subsequently, after outlining these investigations inside the setting of the 24 hours metabolite profiles examined beforehand, the absence of an agreement is maybe to be expected. Indeed, just one of the examinations announced is probably going to have brought about the transcendence of a fasting state throughout 24 hours.

In particular, the investigation investigated the effect of diminishing supper recurrence to one dinner day by day under states of energy balance. Momentarily, fifteen typical weight members finished two 8-week intercession periods in a randomized hybrid plan with a 11-week waste of time stretch. In one treatment, all energy was burned-through in a solitary feast somewhere in the range of 17.00 and 21.00 hours, while the other treatment isolated similar food sources into a regular breakfast, lunch and supper design. To work with consistence, the supper in the two conditions was devoured under oversight and all food varieties were given. The eating regimens were coordinated for both energy and macronutrient content and focused on weight upkeep, with day by day change of recommended admission dependent on body weight estimations, which were then reflected in the contradicting preliminary. No distinctions in weight, body arrangement or wellbeing markers were obvious at the beginning of every treatment and no distinctions in energy consumption, macronutrient balance or active work were noted between the two conditions. Regardless of these invalid discoveries, weight and fat mass (as evaluated by bioelectrical impedance) were decreased by 1.4 and 2.1 kg, separately, following the one feast day by day condition yet not the three suppers every day condition. Notwithstanding, the decrease in adiposity was not joined by upgrades in lipid profile or glycaemia. This is reliable with the earlier idea that expanding the everyday fasting period may bring about expanded use of lipid-inferred substrates in energy digestion and ideal consequences for fat equilibrium.

The up to referenced translation proposes that, similarly as an extended day by day taking care of window might be helpful for an energy excess, drawn out fasting on a standard premise could be a viable technique to counter fat accumulation. Notwithstanding, what is especially intriguing here is that this perception was made under painstakingly coordinated with conditions. While this doesn't bar any chance of some mixture of imperceptible changes in the different segments of energy balance, it is additionally conceivable that the extended fasting period is applying impacts on energy digestion that are autonomous of net energy balance. The current writing on intermittent fasting gives a helpful stage to investigating this thought further.

1.3 Methods

The umbrella term intermittent fasting alludes to a progression of helpful intercessions which target worldly taking care of limitations, ostensibly sorted as: the 5:2 eating regimen, changed substitute day fasting, time-confined taking care of and complete substitute day fasting. Independent of the reasoning for each, such methodologies have been liable to developing prominence as of late, yet test information to help their application are nearly sparse. Obtusely, the quantity of diet books prompting how intermittent fasting can be consolidated into our everyday lives is a few significant degrees more noteworthy than the quantity of logical papers looking at whether intermittent fasting ought to be supported by any means.

Among the most desired types of intermittent fasting is the 5:2 eating routine, wherein extreme energy limitation is forced on 2 d/week with not indispensable utilization on the leftover five. The investigation randomized 63 grown-ups with overweight or heftiness and type 2 diabetes to 12 weeks of either day by day energy limitation or a 5:2 methodology. The 5:2 gathering decreased their admission to 1674–2510 kJ (400–600 kcal) for two non-continuous days out of each week and followed their constant eating regimen on the excess five, while the day by day limitation bunch basically diminished their admission to 5021–6485 kJ (1200–1550 kcal) consistently. Albeit the degree to which remedies were accomplished was not announced, principle impacts of time yet not gathering were seen for decreases in weight, fat mass and without fat mass, just as enhancements in glycated Hb focus and the utilization of diabetic meds. Comparative ends were additionally drawn by two ongoing examinations which thought about this 5:2 methodology (for example 1674–2510 kJ (400–600 kcal) on two non-continuous days out of every week) against day by day energy limitation more than a half year.

This example of results shows a wide equivalency between the metabolic effects of the 5:2 eating regimen and day by day energy limitation, contending against any unique properties of the fasting component as such. Be that as it may, this is certifiably not a reliable finding all through the writing. After looking at the 5:2 methodology (requiring two back to back long periods of 75 % energy limitation each week) against day by day energy limitation (requiring 25 % energy limitation consistently) more than a half year, it is noticed differential changes in fasting insulin and fasting files of insulin opposition. Regardless of comparable decreases in weight and fat mass, the unassuming decreases in fasting insulin and insulin opposition seen in the two gatherings were more articulated with the 5:2 strategy. Albeit this may mirror a more intense impact of utilizing two sequential long periods of extreme energy limitation (instead of non-continuous), there were additionally more prominent decreases in energy and sugar admission in this gathering, which confound the understanding.

Utilizing a comparative methodology, it is looked to think about the impacts of intermittent energy limitation (carried out utilizing the 5:2 methodology) against every day energy limitation when coordinated for net energy equilibrium and along these lines weight misfortunes, to limit the puzzling impact of such factors on metabolic wellbeing. Moreover, this examination highlighted dynamic lists of metabolic control, expanding upon the earlier investigations which just included abstained measures. Momentarily, 27 members with overweight or corpulence were randomized to attempt either an intermittent or a consistent energy limitation diet. The 5:2 condition confined members to 2636 kJ (630 kcal)/d for two sequential days every week, with a self-chose vigorous eating routine on the leftover five. Similarly, the consistent limitation carried out a self-chose diet proposed to lessen energy admission by 2510 kJ (600 kcal)/d. Rather than getting back to the research center after a fixed period, members were rethought after accomplishing a 5 % weight reduction. In spite of bigger decreases in energy consumption in the intermittent condition, the plan implied that adjustments of weight were comparative between gatherings. Body organization and fasting biochemical results were additionally comparatively influenced by the two eating regimens, showing great concurrence with past examinations. Be that as it may, the intermittent eating regimen brought about critical decreases in postprandial TAG focuses comparative with every day energy limitation, while postprandial C-peptide fixation likewise showed an inclination for more noteworthy decreases in the intermittent taking care of gathering. The creators inferred that this features a possible prevalence of intermittent relative over constant energy limitation.

In light of the in advance of referenced investigations of the 5:2 way to deal with intermittent fasting, it appears to be that the way wherein the quick is applied is a critical determinant of the effects on metabolic wellbeing. At the point when the quick is attempted on continuous days, there is an evident prevalence relative over every day energy limitation, while applying the quick on non-successive day's outcomes in extensively comparable impacts. After thinking about this as far as the resultant continuous fasting length, this would seem to fit with the recommendation of Anton et al.(28), as fasting on sequential days is bound to bring about a continuous quick of more than 12–14 hours when contrasted and fasting on non-successive days. In any case, as these mediations don't bind the allowed consumption during fasting to a particular time window (for example 1674–2510 kJ (400–600 kcal) burned-through somewhere in the range of 12.00 and 14.00 hours on fasting days), this makes it hard to build up the specific term of supreme fasting accomplished.

1.4 Modified Alternate-Day Fasting for Normal Weight

Most of human investigations which look at intermittent fasting have focused upon a technique alluded to as adjusted substitute day fasting. It contrasts from the 5:2 eating routine in two key respects: the serious limitation is applied during exchanging days (ostensibly 24 hours, albeit basically more differed to oblige rest); and any allowed energy during fasting is given in a solitary feast (along these lines guaranteeing an unmistakable augmentation of the common short-term quick). A significant part of the work embraced in this field starts from spearheading tests in which members were needed to shift back and forth between 24 hours times of fasting and not obligatory taking care of, with a solitary 2510–3347 kJ (600–800 kcal) supper allowed somewhere in the range of 12.00 and 14.00 hours on non-taking care of days.

The impacts of this methodology on weight were at first investigated in a solitary arm preliminary, where twelve fat members finished two months of changed substitute day fasting. Announced adherence to the fasting convention stayed high all through, with energy admission averaging 26 % of routine. Nearly, consumption on taking care of days came to 95 % of the routine level, coming about in a 37 % net energy limitation by and large. This prompted weight misfortunes of 5.6 kg, 5.4 kg of which was represented by diminishes in fat mass. Complete cholesterol, LDL-cholesterol and TAG were additionally diminished by at any rate 20 %, impacts which were related with upgrades in adipokine profile. Ensuing work by a similar gathering flawlessly exhibits that these results are comparable when applied to accomplices of grown-ups who are overweight, when dinner timing on the fasting day is changed, and that simultaneous macronutrient control doesn't apply added substance impacts.

All in all, these information recommend that adjusted substitute day fasting might be a feasible methods for improving cardio metabolic wellbeing in grown-ups who are overweight or stout. Notwithstanding,

94

without a relative every day energy limitation bunch, it is hard to confine any autonomous impacts of the fasting time frames from the impacts of energy limitation or potentially related weight reduction. This was tended to as of late by an examination of the two strategies under isoenergetic conditions comparative with a no mediation control bunch. Momentarily, 69 grown-ups with heftiness were randomized to attempt a half year of adjusted substitute day fasting or every day energy limitation. The other day fasting diet limited members to a solitary feast containing 25 % of their deliberate energy prerequisites somewhere in the range of 12.00 and 14.00 hours during fasting periods, yet endorsed 125 % of energy necessities on taking care of days. On the other hand, the day by day energy limitation diet endorsed a 25 % decrease in energy consumption consistently, bringing about a comparable decrease in energy admission of 25 % in the two gatherings. Macronutrient balance was protected in the two occasions and the accomplished energy limitation was 21 and 24 % for substitute day fasting and every day energy limitation, separately. The noticed weight deficiency of 6•8 % was likewise comparative between the two gatherings, an example driven by changes in both fat mass and lean mass. Abstained markers of metabolic wellbeing were likewise to a great extent unaffected by one or the other intercession, including lipid profile, provocative markers, adipokines, glucose fixation and insulin opposition. Besides, not many contrasts arose during a following half year weight support period in which the taking care of examples were kept up however the remedies changed to satisfy energy necessities (for example no energy deficiency).

This indeed demonstrates that intermittent fasting and day by day energy limitation apply comparable consequences for most wellbeing results, as closed beforehand for the 5:2 methodology. Be that as it may, during the changed substitute day fasting mediation, members reliably over-burned-through on fasting days and under-burned-through on took care of days, in what the creators portray as true energy limitation. By and large. However when the 34 members that attempted substitute day fasting were separated into the individuals who lost pretty much than 5 % weight, those nearest to the endorsed admission targets showed bigger declines in weight regardless of burning-through more energy overall(69). Tragically, the components supporting this are indistinct. The perception could reflect expanded utilization of lipid-inferred substrates or lower levels of versatile thermogenesis with intermittent techniques, or maybe it just reflects more unfortunate dietary detailing by those with lower adherence.

In any case, information rising up out of investigations of changed substitute day fasting don't imply a prevalence relative over every day energy limitation. Albeit, the utilization of single-arm preliminaries and helpless adherence to fasting solutions leave this inquiry open to additional investigation.

Incidentally, the adherence gives that seem normal to adjusted substitute day approaches may lie in the burden of an extreme limitation instead of a total quick, which in being an outright (though more serious) could truth be told work with consistence. Drawing from this reason, time-limited taking care of is another strategy for intermittent fasting which has arisen as of late and requires no information on food piece or limitation at eating events, just attention to the time at which eating events are allowed by any means. This methodology intends to limit food admission to a transient window (commonly 10 hours) inside the waking stage, along these lines lessening taking care of chances and stretching out the overnight quick to at any rate 14 hours every day.

Work in our research facility investigated the effect of broadening the overnight quick on energy equilibrium and supplement digestion, in this way giving a few bits of knowledge with respect with the impacts of such techniques. At first, 33 grown-ups who were of sound weight were randomized to about a month and a half of either burning-through breakfast, characterized as in any event 2929 kJ (700 kcal) before 11.00 hours every day (with half devoured inside 2 hours of waking), or expanded daytime fasting as of recently. Strangely, upgrades in anthropometric boundaries and fasting wellbeing markers were not genuinely unique between mediations. In arrangement, a board of chemicals embroiled in the guideline of energy balance showed little change following the two intercessions, albeit explicit proportions of fat tissue insulin affectability recommended an improvement in the morning meal bunch as it were.

These to a great extent invalid discoveries comparative with earlier exploration could be clarified by the free-living methodology used to examine compensatory changes in segments of energy balance. The fasting bunch devoured less energy than the morning meal bunch when arrived at the midpoint of all through every 24 hours' time frame, yet this was made up for by lower actual work thermogenesis. After applying this convention to an associate of grown-ups with corpulence, broadened fasting came about in a somewhat more prominent compensatory expansion in energy admission following fasting (albeit still not satisfactory to balance the energy burned-through or overlooked at breakfast), while every day fasting was again causally identified with lower actual work energy consumption in the first part of the day. Strangely, in this accomplice with weight breakfast came about in improved insulinaemic reactions during an oral glucose resilience test comparative with the fasting condition. In any case, this test was adjusted for circadian cycle instead of taking care of cycle, so the noticed finding could essentially reflect better arrangement with expected occasions in the morning meal condition.

Different examinations have applied time-confined taking care of under fiery conditions, similar as the investigation. Zeroing in on energy digestion, it is randomized 34 men to about two months of time-confined taking care of or a control diet. Diets were coordinated for energy and macronutrient substance and intended to give 100 % of energy prerequisites across three dinners in the two conditions. In the control condition, dinners were devoured at 08.00, 13.00 and 20.00 hours, while in the exploratory condition, suppers were burned-through at 13.00, 16.00 and 20.00 hours to allow a 16 hours quick. The time-confined methodology brought about decreases in fat mass comparative with controls, which were banded together by diminishes in RER, showing a shift towards fat oxidation. Strangely, notwithstanding, in spite of going with decreases in leptin and hypothalamic–pituitary–thyroid flagging, resting energy consumption was kept up. This supports the thought that supplement timing impacts upon supplement digestion, while likewise featuring that this seems to happen indeed with a 16 hours quick comparative with a 12 hours quick. Considering this considering the common postprandial supplement profile talked about already, the expansion in fasting span may give more freedoms to the digestion of substrates got from endogenous lipids. This again focuses to the likelihood that standard augmentation of the fasting time frame past 12–14 hours might be vital to these advantages, which was not really accomplished by the 5:2 or adjusted substitute day techniques talked about before. The essential inquiry is whether these upgrades are improved with significantly longer spans of complete fasting.

More delayed and complete fasting was as of late analyzed by analysts, who guessed that circadian rhythms in energy digestion would potentiate the impacts of time-limited taking care of when eating times are bound to before phases of the waking stage. Utilizing a rehashed measures hybrid plan, they thought about the impact of devouring all day by day energy inside a 6 hours window and a 12 hours window more than 5 weeks in men with pre-diabetes. The weight control plans were endorsed dependent on energy prerequisites to keep up energy balance and were likewise coordinated for energy and macronutrient content. Consistence to the two conditions was high and the all-encompassing fasting period was joined by decreases in fasting insulin, top insulin and insulin opposition during an oral glucose resilience test. Be that as it may, it seems the extent and determination of any treatment impacts may have required a more drawn out wash-out span between rehashed medicines, as the effects on insulinaemia were apparently influenced by standard contrasts emerging from a preliminary request impact. Joined with the way that the fasting term going before post-mediation estimations was not normalized across preliminaries, further examinations are justified to check these captivating prospects.

In light of all the up to referenced discoveries, the proof focuses with an impact of expanded fasting stretches on fat mass free of energy balance, especially when the fasting span is reached out to in any event 16 hours, as demonstrated by specialists. In the two cases, this created critical decreases in fat mass comparative with a standard 12 hours quick, which ensnares expanded fasting past 12 hours as a key factor. Be that as it may, the significance of such changes for metabolic wellbeing is less clear because of a progression of puzzling impacts.

1.6 Complete alternate-day fasting for Over Weight

So far, the intermittent fasting techniques talked about ordinarily license the utilization of energy inside every 24 hours cycle somewhat, implying that the fasting stretch is just reached out by a couple of hours. This is principally to work with adherence yet it additionally recharges hepatic glycogen stores and lessens the usage of lipid-determined substrates (for example ketone bodies), which may veil a few proposed advantages of intermittent fasting. Moreover, this interruption is significantly topsy-turvy, in that even a short taking care of event quickly smothers lipolysis and ketogenesis, which at that point don't return for various hours. It is deserving of note at this point that the consideration of actual work or exercise during the abstained period may serve to speed up the rebuilding of these pathways somewhat, albeit the simultaneous utilization of intermittent fasting close by practice intercessions is past the extent of this audit. Regardless, the 20 hours fasting span utilized by specialist is probably going to have prompted a more noteworthy dependence on these lipid-determined substrates throughout 24 hours, which may clarify the decrease in fat mass notwithstanding enthusiastic admission.

Expanding upon this reason, it is applied a 20 hours quick on substitute days from 22.00 to 18.00 hours, addressing a combination of the methodologies utilized by researchers. Fasting precluded all admission except for water, while during the mediating taking care of periods, members were advised to twofold their ongoing admission to keep up weight. Albeit dietary admission was not checked, blood tests gathered in a subset of fasting periods affirmed consistence with the fasting convention, with comparing changes in foundational groupings of glucose, glycerol, adiponectin and leptin. Albeit both weight and fat mass were unaltered, the glucose imbuement rate during an euglycaemic–hyperinsulinaemic cinch expanded in the last 30 minutes of the testing time frame, proposing upgraded insulin affectability following total substitute day fasting. Appropriately, this was joined by more fast concealment of fat tissue lipolysis during the insulin imbuement. While the absence of an impact on weight and fat mass comparative with earlier examinations may mirror the uniqueness in total fasting time, the creators were regardless ready to reason that this way to deal with intermittent fasting can improve metabolic wellbeing even without perceptible changes in weight.

Utilizing a comparative methodology, selected eight guys of sound load to a rehashed measures hybrid investigation. This looked at the impacts of about fourteen days of a standard weight upkeep diet against about fourteen days of an intermittent fasting diet, utilizing a similar fasting convention. In this example, a more prescriptive methodology was embraced to the taking care of cycles, with fluid suppers used to reinforce admission and change of solutions in case of significant weight change. As needs be, weight and piece were unaltered, yet there were no huge changes in glucose, lipid or protein energy in the basal state, or during a two-stage euglycaemic–hyperinsulinaemic brace. In reality, the solitary distinction was a slight abatement in resting energy use following the intermittent fasting arm.

In spite of the investigations of scientists, the in advance of referenced discoveries propose that intermittent expansion of the fasting time frame applies no impact on energy or supplement digestion, beside a potential decrease in resting energy use. While there are a few inconsistencies as far as the way to deal with taking care of cycles and appraisal of supplement digestion under unique conditions, crediting to such factors would propose the impact is probably not going to be clinically significant. Notwithstanding, work by Heilbronn et al. gives intriguing bits of knowledge that could clarify such obvious differences between apparently comparative methodologies. Their investigation applied an intermittent fasting mediation to an associate of sixteen grown-ups who were not fat which included fasting from one 12 PM to another on rotating days for 3 weeks, with fasting periods just allowing without energy beverages and sans sugar gum (took care of periods were not obligatory). Evaluations of body arrangement, a blended dinner test and muscle biopsies were completed at pattern and follow-up, with an extra arrangement of estimations gathered following a 36 hours quick to investigate the physiological effect of individual fasting periods on energy digestion.

Despite the fact that energy admission was not detailed, the mediation diminished weight by 2.5 %, around 66% of which was represented by decreased fat mass. Be that as it may, most of fasting boundaries, including plasma glucose focus, RMR, substrate oxidation and muscle GLUT4 content showed no remarkable change. Key exemptions were sex-explicit changes in cholesterol profile, with ladies encountering an expansion in HDL-cholesterol focus and men showing decreases in fasting TAG. Qualities gathered following a day and a half of fasting affirmed expanded unsaturated fat oxidation, bringing up the issue of why the everyday practice up-guideline of fat digestion joined with weight misfortunes brought about no reliable changes in metabolic wellbeing. Be that as it may, this example of sexual dimorphism proceeded into postprandial results, with expansions in glucose region under bend for females and decreases in insulin region under bend for guys.

It may then be recommended that guys and females react contrastingly to finish substitute day fasting. Notwithstanding, there were various standard contrasts among people in that review which ought to be considered in this understanding, with men showing higher glucose, insulin and TAG fixations in the abstained state. After contextualizing this in the physiology of insulin resistance(9–14), it appears to be conceivable that the metabolic condition of male members at pattern may remain to profit more from the standard augmentation of fasting (despite the chance of measurable relapse). In these people, the shift toward fat oxidation found in light of delayed fasting could assist with clearing lipid mediators from non-fat tissues, in this way improving insulin affectability. This is upheld by the announced expansion in carnitine palmitoltransferase-1 protein content in muscle tissue after the intercession.

Stretching out this reason to the investigations of scientists, the normal muscle to fat ratio of their accomplices was 20.1 and 14.8 %, separately. This may along these lines support the thought that those with lower levels of adiposity may not profit by such mediations. Subsequently, it is basic to consider the apparently particular reactions seen among less fatty and more overweight partners when deciphering the aftereffects of comparable investigations. This isn't simply because the potential for weight reduction and wellbeing gain may shift, yet in addition on the grounds that the show as lean or hefty at standard might be indicative of an inclination towards different compensatory changes that anticipate responsiveness to treatment.

Facilitating this line of enquiry, embraced a randomized controlled preliminary of complete substitute day fasting in an example of grown-ups with corpulence. Momentarily, 26 members were randomized to attempt two months of either every day energy limitation (requiring a decrease in energy admission of 1674 kJ (400 kcal)/d) or a total substitute day quick. The intermittent fasting condition forced a quick on each and every other day and gave an eating regimen to meet assessed day by day energy necessities during taking care of periods, with a progression of 837 kJ (200 kcal) discretionary food modules to allow not indispensable admission. All food sources were given and diets were coordinated to macronutrient balance instead of energy consumption. Thusly, energy consumption across the mediation was lower with the intermittent fasting approach, averaging 53 % of weight support prerequisites contrasted and 72 % for every day energy limitation. This was joined by a pattern for more prominent decreases in weight with intermittent fasting comparative with energy limitation, with 8.8 and 6.2 % decreases found in the separate conditions. In spite of this, fat mass and lean mass diminished to a comparable degree in the two gatherings, an example reflected by upgrades in abstained lipid profile. Just intermittent fasting created upgrades in abstained glucose focus from gauge to follow-up, yet reactions to a powerful trial of insulin affectability were unaltered. Alternately, RMR was diminished by day by day energy limitation just, following amendment for body piece changes, with a pattern for a between-bunch contrast. Be that as it may, between-bunch examinations were undermined by pattern contrasts, with those in the day by day energy limitation bunch giving higher weight and fasting insulin fixations all things considered.

1.7 Summary

Intermittent fasting plainly includes a wide range of dietary mediations. The characterizing trademark is the imprisonment of energy limitation to a predetermined transient window, be that 16 hours every day, each and every other day or only 2 days of the week. Across these different models, intermittent fasting can inspire decreases in weight and upgrades in metabolic wellbeing, impacts which show up extensively equivalent to standard every day energy limitation. In any case, on the grounds that the remedial capability of these worldly systems may lie in regularly broadening catabolic periods, consequently expanding dependence on lipid-determined substrates, the comparable adequacy corresponding to standard methodologies could rather mirror an inability to seriously broaden the post-absorptive period. The 5:2 eating regimen and changed substitute day fasting infrequently exclude more than one supper in arrangement and consequently this progress to lipid-determined substrates may barely be made. Then again, if applying approaches that expand the fasting span towards 20 h and past (for example sequential fasting days in the 5:2 eating routine or time-limited taking care of), this progress to lipid-inferred substrates is probably going to be made all the more every now and again, maybe clarifying the proposed predominance of these methodologies. Lamentably, while the last investigations of complete substitute day fasting offer among the longest continuous fasting time frames, the genuine impacts of this are hard to disengage because of metabolically different examples and the utilization of single-arm preliminaries. Thusly, there stays an earnest requirement for all around planned, randomized-controlled preliminaries of this ordinarily received methodology.

1.8 Future directions

Distinguishing more powerful methodologies for overseeing stoutness and related metabolic problems stays a general wellbeing challenge and intermittent fasting may address an intense apparatus. Notwithstanding, exploration to help this is scant and various significant features have been ignored. Further examination is in this manner justified to build up whether intermittent fasting is essentially an elective methods for accomplishing energy limitation, or a dietary methodology which offers an ideal technique for keeping up/improving metabolic wellbeing.

Body composition

While much examination has been given with the impacts intermittent fasting applies on fat equilibrium, regularly expanding catabolic periods additionally conveys suggestions for without fat mass. Scientists contend that the expanded dependence on lipid-determined substrates during delayed fasting serves to limit disintegrations in bulk and capacity, albeit this doesn't invalidate these weakening altogether. Unthinkingly, net protein balance is a result of steady communications between protein blend and breakdown. Following an overnight quick (roughly 8–12 hours), there is an expansion in amino corrosive efflux from muscle tissue, recommending a change for net muscle protein breakdown. While there are restricted information to help a distortion of this catabolic state when the fasting term is reached out to 24 hours, a new report showed that fasting for 72 hours multiplied the pace of amino corrosive efflux from skeletal muscle when contrasted and a 10 hours quick. As needs be, it is sensible to expect a more prominent decrease in sans fat mass in light of intermittent fasting when contrasted and day by day energy limitation.

As opposed to this unthinking viewpoint, nonetheless, a methodical audit of randomized-controlled preliminaries inferred that intermittent fasting may truth be told offer upgraded maintenance of sans fat mass when contrasted and day by day energy limitation. A comparative end was additionally drawn by a later audit contrasting intermittent methodologies and low energy eating less junk food. While the prevalence of adjusted substitute day fasting concentrates in the previous survey may assist with clarifying this, it is deserving of note that the total substitute day investigations of scientists were incorporated. Whenever checked, improved maintenance of without fat mass comparative with day by day energy limitation would be a strong resource thinking about its relationship with RMR. Thus, explaining the impact of complete substitute day fasting on sans fat mass ought to be a focal examination need.

Energy Expenditure

A key (however regularly neglected) issue with customary corpulence the executives approaches is compensatory changes in different elements of energy balance, especially diminished energy consumption with day by day energy limitation. It isn't obvious from the current group of intermittent fasting research whether such compensatory changes might be summoned. Zeroing in at first on RMR, the two scientists detailed no noticeable change in light of complete substitute day fasting, specialists recommend a decrease in resting energy utilization of 247 kJ (59 kcal)/d. On the other hand, active work energy consumption has not been altogether and unbiasedly analyzed because of complete substitute day fasting. It is noticed no progressions in every day step tallies during about two months of adjusted substitute day fasting, notwithstanding clinically significant weight misfortunes, and following investigations utilizing accelerometers have checked this result. Notwithstanding, it ought to be noticed that these investigations all utilized adjusted substitute day fasting draws near, which can sensibly be required to contrast in their impacts on deliberate conduct comparative with complete substitute day techniques.

Without target proportions of energy consumption, specialist contend that energy use isn't influenced by transient limitations of energy admission dependent on the shortfall of huge contrasts in weight in their vigorous time-confined taking care of study. Notwithstanding, specialist feature that precise assurance of energy balance requires estimation of all parts of the condition. While it does then stay a particular chance that run of the mill compensatory reactions to an energy shortfall are blunted when intermittent fasting, an absence of proof about disengaged measurements of energy use at present forestalls solid ends being drawn. There is in this way a distinct need to analyze the total effect of intermittent fasting on the parts of energy balance in a solid and all around controlled way, not least active work thermogenesis.

Postprandial Nutrient Metabolism

A chance emerging from the prior writing comes from the way that most of studies have zeroed in on fasting proportions of glucose, insulin and TAG, with not very many examinations utilizing dynamic tests. The significance of this is very much represented by the effect of intermittent fasting on insulin; upgrades in fasting insulin have been reliably appeared in various investigations as explored by analysts. They likewise show that in a subset of these investigations, fasting lists of insulin opposition, for example, the homeostasis model for the most part improve following a time of intermittent fasting. Nonetheless, it is imperative to take note of that while these fasting records are valuable in facilitating test requests, there are a few constraints. For example, analyst propose it is feasible for a member to be insulin safe without showing fasting hyperinsulinaemia.

Similar intermittententities arise while looking at postprandial glycaemia, while postprandial lipaemia has been generally overlooked. On an intense premise, scientist show that daily of 100 % vigorous limitation brings about upgraded concealment of postprandial TAG and NEFA fixations, comparative with routine admission and halfway energy limitation. Stretching out this to the 5:2 methodology, a comparative example arose for upgrades in postprandial TAG fixations with the intermittent condition comparative with consistent limitation. Such impacts are likewise predictable with the improved concealment of fat tissue lipolysis announced. Given the significance of these results with regards to heftiness and the related comorbidities, closer assessment is justified.

Comparative Designs

In spite of being proposed as an elective way to deal with weight reduction, not many human preliminaries to date have straightforwardly analyzed total substitute day fasting against standard day by day energy limitation. Despite the fact that it is for the most part announced that the results are comparative, the expansive range of companions and trial conventions utilized puzzles solid examinations against the previous writing. The investigation is unquestionably an exemption for this example, as they straightforwardly analyzed total substitute day fasting and day by day energy limitation; nonetheless, the two conditions were not coordinated for the level of energy limitation forced. Hence, arriving at an agreement on the general benefits of intermittent fasting is beyond the realm of imagination minus any additional investigations with fitting controls.

Fasting-Dependent Effects

In conclusion, and maybe in particular, is the likelihood that excess in a post-absorptive state for delayed periods (for example fasting) may grant autonomous medical advantages past the set up impacts of the net negative energy balance fundamentally (and hence weight reduction). This is upheld who propose critical upgrades in insulin affectability because of complete substitute day fasting; yet the inability to recreate this finding with a close to indistinguishable fasting convention renders current information obscure. This contention might be driven by methodological differences in benchmark adiposity and the re-taking care of convention utilized, however it leaves a relevant inquiry regardless. In the event that fasting-subordinate consequences for wellbeing do exist, are traditional dinner designs adding to metabolic unsettling influences independent of energy content? This would imply that adjustments of taking care of times could establish a novel element of what is viewed as a solid eating regimen, instead of just being a vehicle for energy limitation.

In basic terms, nourishing contemplations can be comprehensively characterized under the three headings of type, amount and timing, with current dietary rules, for example, the guide giving an unmistakable and confirmed representation of the initial two classes (for example what food sources we ought to eat and the amount we ought to eat). Further exploration is expected to finish the image and incorporate proposals about when we ought to eat; or decide not to.

Chapter 2: Effect of Intermittent Fasting Programs on Body Composition

Intermittent fasting (IF) envelops an assortment of explicit projects that utilization momentary diets to improve body creation and in general wellbeing through adjusted substrate use and hormonal changes. This survey looks at the impacts of IF programs on body arrangement and talks about possible ramifications for competitors, especially those contending in weight-confined games. Intermittent fasting can diminish body weight and muscle to fat ratio in non-competitors, however little is known with respect to athletic populaces. Blended outcomes in regards to maintenance of sans fat mass have additionally been accounted for. A conversation of how data from the current writing can be circumspectly utilized for application in weight-confined competitors is given.

2.1 Introduction

Competitors and dynamic people frequently look to improve their body synthesis by expanding bulk with insignificant fat addition or by diminishing muscle versus fat while keeping up existing bulk. A mix of activity and wholesome mediations is normally prescribed to seek after these objectives. Inside athletic populaces, accomplishing a low muscle to fat ratio is especially significant for those contending in weight-confined or "body arrangement delicate" sports like blended combative techniques, boxing, wrestling, aerobatic, rock climbing, and figure skating. For battle competitors attempting to shed pounds, the most widely recognized dietary system is restricting every day caloric admission with the goal that caloric utilization is not exactly the sum expected to keep up existing body weight. To accomplish this objective of day by day caloric limitation, a few dietary methodologies are usually utilized by people trying to get more fit like eating more modest and more successive suppers for the duration of the day, restricting carb utilization, restricting fat admission, and expanding protein consumption. Notwithstanding, day by day caloric limitation can be hard to keep up throughout significant stretches of time.

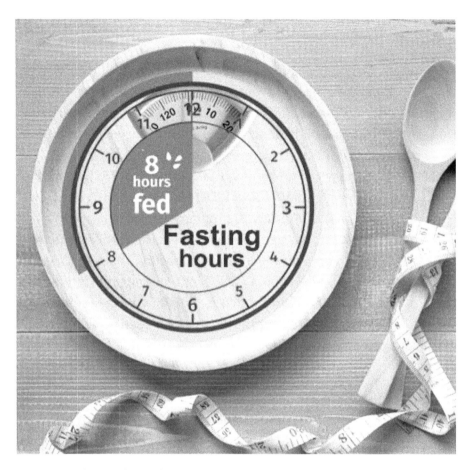

In weight-limited battle sports like boxing and blended combative techniques, it isn't unprecedented for competitors to lose moderately a lot of body weight before rivalry. After rivalry, huge measures of weight are frequently recaptured in view of the trouble of keeping a specific dietary system. On the off chance that this occurs, battle competitors may endeavor to depend on quicker, and possibly dangerous, weight reduction systems to plan for ensuing rivalries. This may include losing a lot of "water weight" long before their authority "say something" or rivalry, which can antagonistically influence execution and prosperity. Consequently, battle competitors specifically may profit by a dietary system that could hypothetically be kept up consistently and conceivably limit huge irritations in weight between rivalries. This may moderate the need to lose so much "water weight" paving the way to rivalry, subsequently permitting a possibly less troublesome and more secure weight cut.

Intermittent fasting (IF) is one possible system important to weight-limited competitors. In the event that utilizations normal transient diets fully intent on improving body structure and in general wellbeing. Despite the fact that IF is an expansive term that envelops various explicit projects, most structures can be separated into the accompanying classes: time-confined taking care of (TRF), substitute day fasting (ADF), entire day fasting (WDF), and Ramadan IF. It is critical to take note of that numerous IF programs utilize adjusted fasting instead of genuine fasting. Genuine fasting requires forbearance from all caloric admission, however altered fasting permits modest quantities of caloric admission. In any event, during adjusted fasting, the absolute energy burned-through is definitely lower than weight support energy needs. Adjusted fasting can be seen as following an extremely low–calorie diet however just on specific days or parts of days.

Time-limited intermittent fasting diet for fat misfortune, muscle gain and wellbeing. Accessible from some source normally comprises of following a similar eating design every day, with specific hours containing the fasting time frame (12–20 hours) and the leftover hours including the taking care of window. There is fluctuation between programs in the arrangement of the fasting and taking care of periods during the day, yet it is generally basic to put the taking care of period in the evening. Substitute day fasting switches back and forth between not obligatory taking care of days (i.e., unhindered eating) and pseudo fasting days that permit 1 feast containing 25% of every day calorie needs. Entire day fasting (e.g., Eat Stop Eat) comprises of 1–2 days of fasting each week and not obligatory eating on different days.

Ramadan IF is basically a strict quick instead of a fasting routine utilized explicitly to improve body piece and wellbeing. The impacts of Ramadan on body structure and athletic execution have been recently summed up and won't be the focal point of this survey. It is imperative to take note of that both food and liquid admission are confined during Ramadan. The expected effect of lack of hydration and modified rest plans during Ramadan make understanding and use of these investigations more troublesome.

Albeit most of the exploration to date has not been led with an athletic populace, the current collection of proof exhibits possible advantages and worries of IF projects and makes way for future investigations in competitors. The reason for this survey is to examine the current exploration in the domain of IF, especially consequences for body weight and creation, and to talk about its possible appropriateness as an elective dietary methodology for competitors contending in weight-confined games.

2.2 Metabolic Changes of Fasting

During momentary fasting, a progress in substrate use happens, which diminishes dependence on carb and builds dependence on unsaturated fats. Despite the fact that blood glucose levels decrease, entire body lipolysis and fat oxidation increment all through the initial 24 hours of food hardship. The time span somewhere in the range of 18 and 24 hours of fasting has shown a half diminishing in glucose oxidation and a half expansion in fat oxidation. It is believed that expanded thoughtful sensory system action, higher groupings of development chemical, and decreased insulin focuses may add to this change in substrate use.

One concern related with fasting is that muscle will be catabolized to give substrate to gluconeogenesis. It is realized that people adjust to delayed starvation by monitoring body protein, yet expanded proteolysis has been seen during momentary fasting contemplates. In any case, most of these examinations looked at estimations taken after an overnight quick with those required 60+ hours after the fact. Since the length of diets during mainstream IF conventions is a lot more limited than 60 hours (e.g., as long as 24 hours), it is conceivable that bulk misfortune doesn't happen in a similar way during more limited diets.

Early writing analyzing total fasting detailed that protein catabolism didn't start to increment until the third day of fasting, and tracked down that fourteen days of ADF (switching back and forth between 20-hour fasting and 28-hour taking care of) didn't change entire body protein digestion in slender sound men. Albeit these metabolic changes are fascinating, it ought to be noticed that the impacts of ongoing momentary diets might be not the same as brief times of transient fasting in people who regularly follow a typical eating design. Studies that explicitly analyze IF conventions and track changes in body arrangement are the best proof with respect to the viability of these projects.

118

Entire day fasting regularly comprises of 1 or 2 days of complete or adjusted fasting every week. Entire day fasting contemplates have detailed decreases of 3–9% in body weight, just as diminished muscle to fat ratio mass. No adjustment of lean mass was seen in 3 of the investigations, however it is accounted for a 1% decline following 12 weeks of WDF. Two investigations didn't report changes in lean mass. A limit of these examinations is that just one utilized DXA to assess changes in body creation, while the rest of BIA. It presents an outline of the strategies and aftereffects of WDF examines. In spite of ADF, most WDF considers have analyzed exclusively male or female subjects, instead of a mix. Be that as it may, in view of the contrasts between test plan and subjects utilized (i.e., ordinary weight and overweight guys versus fat females), it is absurd to expect to decide sex contrasts in the reactions to these projects as of now.

At the point when Ramadan IF considers are prohibited, there is almost no examination looking at TRF programs. Specialists led an investigation of TRF, which utilized day by day 20-hour diets in male and female members. The examination utilized a randomized get over plan with two 8-week times of eating either 1 dinner each day or 3 suppers each day. These 2 stages were isolated by 11-week waste of time period, and all food was given to the subjects all through the investigation. During the 1 feast each day stage, members burned-through the entirety of their calories inside a 4-hour window of time in the evening. In the wake of eating 1 supper each day, as contrasted and 3 dinners each day, lower-body weight and fat mass were accounted for. Albeit the two medicines were intended to be isocaloric, the subjects ate 65 less calories each day during the 1 dinner each day period of the examination due to "outrageous completion" and trouble eating all the food in the assigned time window. It is conceivable that people would have eaten even less in the event that they had been allowed to pick when to quit eating, and a lower level of energy admission might have prompted much more prominent weight reduction. The capacity to hold fast to this kind of eating design is problematic, as shown by higher appraisals of appetite and want to eat in the 1 feast each day bunch. The seriousness of these marvels expanded all through the investigation, showing that the subjects didn't become enough used to the eating design.

It is additionally revealed a pattern (p is equivalent to 0.06) for more noteworthy without fat mass in the wake of devouring 1 feast each day (50.9 kg) than subsequent to burning-through 3 suppers each day (49.4 kg). It ought to be noticed that body creation was evaluated utilizing BIA, which has been recently addressed concerning sans fat mass estimations during fasting. Scientist inspected non-hefty people going through a total quick for 43 days (subjects just ingested water, nutrients, and electrolytes). During the later phases of fasting (between the 31st and 43rd day), BIA detailed unreasonable expansions in without fat mass, and the creators expressed that these discoveries should be dismissed as a result of problematic credibility. In any case, the fasting conventions utilized by analysts changed impressively. Subjects in the investigation didn't go through complete fasting for even 1 whole day, and the dietary changes made were not close to as outrageous as those in the examination. Taken together, these examinations may show that BIA isn't the ideal device for estimating lean mass changes during such fasting conventions, and the pattern for more prominent sans fat mass announced by specialist ought to be deciphered warily.

No activity intercession was utilized in the investigation, and no progressions in active work were found throughout the examination. It ought to be noticed that there was a 28.6% withdrawal rate from the investigation, demonstrating that a few people will be unable to cling to this example of eating. Notwithstanding, there is restricted long haul achievement of keeping up weight reduction instigated by a day by day hypo caloric eating routine.

As far as anyone is concerned, just one investigation has inspected joining an IF convention with an activity program. The examination analyzed 4 gatherings: ADF, ADF in addition to work out, practice alone, and control. Twelve weeks of directed perseverance practice on fixed bicycles and circular machines was executed in the 2 practicing gatherings. Subjects practiced 3 times each week, starting with 25 minutes at 60% of their age-anticipated greatest pulse (HRmax) and advancing to 40 minutes at 75% HRmax throughout the span of the examination. It was not revealed whether subjects practiced on altered fasting days or on not indispensable taking care of days, just as whether subjects practiced in an abstained or took care of state.

The ADF in addition to practice bunch lost more weight and fat mass than some other gathering. The ADF and exercise alone gatherings both shed pounds and fat mass yet didn't contrast in the sum lost. There were no contrasts between bunches for sans fat mass changes, albeit the ADF showed a little lessening in without fat mass. Lean mass was held in the gathering that practiced and followed ADF, and the creators revealed that the activity program may have been mindful. A constraint of this investigation is that BIA was utilized to quantify body structure.

Supper recurrence is frequently a polarizing theme, and numerous wellness experts suggest a moderately high dinner recurrence. Albeit the quantity of studies explicitly looking at changed IF conventions is restricted, examinations of feast recurrence adjustments can give some extra data about impacts of diminishing dinner recurrence.

In 1997, analyst basically inspected the writing to survey whether there are advantages of expanding supper recurrence to decrease body weight. They reasoned that epidemiological proof for these advantages is exceptionally feeble. They additionally distinguished 2 significant issues with observational investigations of dinner recurrence and weight acquire: post hoc changes in supper recurrence after weight gain and distorting of energy admission. The post hoc changes happen when people skip dinners to keep up or get thinner after weight acquire has effectively happened, producing a fake opposite connection between supper recurrence and body weight. Distorting of energy admission is very much archived, and information from NHANES I Epidemiological Follow-Up Study highlight inescapable underreporting of food consumption, especially by the individuals who are overweight and announced low dinner frequencies. In the NHANES information, detailed energy admission shows a reverse relationship with weight file and skinfold thickness that seems, by all accounts, to be puzzling separated from underreporting of energy consumption.

The ends came to by specialist were generally repeated in 2011 through a refreshed audit on dinner recurrence by analyst who reasoned that albeit some observational investigations support an opposite connection between body weight and feast recurrence, the larger part don't uphold this (in typical weight, overweight, and corpulent subjects). Notwithstanding the blended outcomes and possible issues in with observational examinations, it was inferred that most of the trial considers neglect to track down any predictable enhancements in body weight or body piece through higher supper frequencies. It likewise gives the idea that the thermic impact of taking care of is unaltered by changes in feast recurrence, albeit a few investigations have shown increments or diminishes in light of lower dinner frequencies. All the more critically, the proof demonstrates that there is no adjustment of 24-hour energy consumption after modifications in feast recurrence going from 2 to 7 suppers each day.

As of late, scientist directed a meta-investigation assessing trial exploration of dinner recurrence as it identifies with body structure. Albeit the underlying consequences of the investigation appeared to support expanded supper recurrence for enhancements in body piece, an affectability examination uncovered that a solitary report was answerable for this outcome. The creators reasoned that if any advantages to sequential feast frequencies exist, they are probably going to be irrelevant as far as commonsense importance, and individual decision ought to generally direct the determination of a dinner recurrence to upgrade consistence.

It ought to be noticed that the line between diminished supper recurrence and IF conventions is to some degree obscured. Intermittent fasting, by definition, is a deliberate decrease in feast recurrence. Nonetheless, IF stresses expanding times of fasting or altered fasting, which isn't really the situation when feast recurrence is generally diminished. For instance, an eating routine that decreases feast recurrence may incorporate suppers at breakfast and supper, which prompts an essentially more limited daytime fasting window (6–10 hours) than a large portion of the IF conventions use. As examined, this drawn out fasting window may effect lipolysis and lipid oxidation, which might actually prompt improved fat misfortune.

The absence of examination explicitly looking at the impacts of executing IF programs in competitors makes it hard to give substantial proposals to the utilization of these projects in competitors. Be that as it may, a few focuses merit considering. Intermittent fasting can be a viable methods for lessening calorie consumption, body weight, and muscle versus fat in non-competitors. Intermittent fasting projects can be intended to permit satisfactory supplement utilization when active work (i.e., practice doesn't need to be acted in an abstained state when an IF program is carried out). A few IF programs are just about as basic as going without food after supper and not having again until breakfast or lunch the following day. These milder TRF programs lead to a time of fasting that is 12–16 hours in term.

Most types of IF could be adjusted to fit a competitor's preparation plan. In ADF and WDF, the changed fasting days comprising of extremely low-energy admission could be utilized less as often as possible or put on rest days or days with lighter preparing exercises. A TRF timetable could be fostered that permits the competitor to eat at the most crucial occasions (e.g., when instructional meetings and rivalry). In any event, utilizing a solitary day out of each seven day stretch of adjusted fasting could assist a competitor with accomplishing a negative energy balance for the week while not upsetting the standard example of food consumption on heavier preparing and rivalry days. In spite of the fact that there is meager proof to show the capacity to cling to these kinds of dietary mediations long haul, IF may give an elective system to competitors who are attempting to get in shape or forestall weight acquire.

Intermittent fasting conventions might be especially material for competitors contending in weight-confined games like blended combative techniques, boxing, and wrestling. These games regularly expect competitors to lose huge measures of weight before rivalry. After rivalry, it isn't extraordinary for these competitors to rapidly recover the weight, making a "yo-yo" example of weight reduction and weight acquire—a cycle that is generally regular in battle sports. Intermittent fasting conventions may give the competitors in these games an elective technique where they couldn't just accomplish week by week caloric shortfalls and weight reduction yet in addition keep up sufficient admission expected to give energy to difficult preparing days.

Presently, there is a scarcity of writing on the impacts of IF conventions on practice execution. In this way, it can't be definitively finished up if these kinds of dietary procedures frustrate or upgrade practice execution, on the off chance that they influence execution by any means. Notwithstanding, if this kind of dietary technique is utilized in a moderate style as depicted here (i.e., fasting one select day of the week or on non-preparing days), it could hypothetically assume a minor part in practice execution in light of the restricted effect on most preparing days. Nonetheless, more exploration and observational information are expected to make more complete ends around here.

It ought to likewise be noticed that there are information showing the significance of routinely burning-through dietary protein to keep up fit muscle tissue, which is a thing of worry for some competitors. Subsequently, this ought to be viewed as when utilizing longer span diets. Scientists have detailed that ingesting 20 grams of whey protein at standard spans at regular intervals might be better in respect than net protein equilibrium and protein amalgamation when contrasted and burning-through a similar aggregate sum of protein (80 grams) in bigger, less incessant or in more modest, more successive dosages. The advantage of eating protein in this amount and recurrence might be expected to the "leucine edge" that is expected to improve protein combination above gauge levels. Consequently, if a competitor utilizes an IF convention, the person in question may decide to adjust it and devour whey protein or another protein source at metered focuses all through the fasting window, especially if lean mass safeguarding is a significant concern.

Future examination explicitly inspecting IF programs in competitors ought to be led, especially in competitors contending in weight-confined games. The fleeting connection between supplement admission and athletic exercises ought to be thought of, and any IF program carried out in athletic populaces should think about the particular prerequisites of the game just as individual variety and inclinations.

Intermittent fasting (IF) is a generally polished dietary strategy that includes intermittent limitation of food utilization. Because of its defensive advantages against metabolic illnesses, maturing, and cardiovascular and neurodegenerative infections, IF keeps on acquiring consideration as a protection and helpful mediation to check these constant sicknesses. Albeit various creature considers have announced positive medical advantages of IF, its possibility and viability in clinical settings stay disputable. Critically, since dietary intercessions, for example, IF have foundational impacts, altogether researching the tissue-explicit changes in creature models is significant to recognize IF's system and assess its likely antagonistic impacts in people. All things considered, we will audit and analyze the results and hidden components of IF in both creature and human investigations. Besides, the impediments of IF and intermittentities among preclinical and clinical investigations will be talked about to give knowledge into the holes between making an interpretation of examination from seat to bedside.

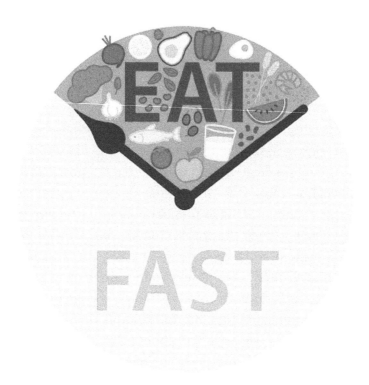

3.1 Introduction

With heftiness rates increasing around the world, it is getting progressively more essential to uncover novel, yet doable, weight-the executives draws near. Because of promising outcomes in preclinical models, different dietary regimens, like intermittent fasting (IF) and caloric limitation (CR), have acquired fame in working with weight reduction and intervening entire body metabolic upgrades. On the off chance that is portrayed by occasional patterns of fasting that can be acted in the presence or the shortfall of caloric decrease. The term incorporates different nourishing systems and eating procedures, for example, time-confined taking care of (TRF), substitute day fasting (ADF), and fasting-copying diet (FMD). TRF alludes to the limitation of energy admission during explicit time spans for the duration of the day;

128

for example, a 16:8 eating regimen incorporates 16 h of fasting with 8-hours eating window. Nearly, ADF is a more thorough eating regimen frequently carried out in clinical settings and requires rotating eating and fasting days, during which people may go through complete fasting or devour an insignificant caloric admission (typically 25% of energy prerequisite during fasting days). Besides, there are varieties of IF regimens, for example, 5:2 or 2:1, which incorporate fasting days consistently. 5:2 IF contains 5 days of taking care of and 2 days of fasting each week (continuously or non-successively). Similarly, 2:1 IF includes 2 days of typical eating followed by 1 day of fasting. This routine furnishes abstained subject with adequate chance to make up for the energy shortage following 1 day of fasting. Hence, 2:1 routine is considered as isocaloric IF in mouse examines. Last, FMD is a low-calorie, low-sugar, low-protein, high-fat eating routine that impersonates the physiological impacts of fasting. These different fasting regimens can fuse CR (which includes decrease of caloric admission) as well as changes in diet synthesis during their eating days to improve the metabolic advantages from the dietary intercessions.

In the event that has been related with different medical advantages, for example, weight the board, expanded life span, improved psychological capacity, decreased oxidative harm, and improved cardiovascular digestion. Albeit numerous investigations exhibiting expanded life span were led in brief life forms like yeast, nematodes, and flies, mammalian model frameworks, especially subject models, have better clarified the physiological ramifications of IF on entire body digestion and tissue-explicit impacts.

These promising medical advantages have accumulated interest from the general population and established researchers, inducing better comprehension of the components by which they improve metabolic intermittentities. In this article, we audit IF concentrates in subjects and people to give understanding into the foundational impacts of IF, and examine its likely ramifications in clinical settings.

In the event that has been viewed as a mediation with benefits past weight reduction. It is because of these promising outcomes that the possibility of IF is altogether researched inside clinical settings. Various investigations have detailed the beneficial outcomes of IF in body-weight and fat-mass decrease, improved glucose homeostasis, and diminished corpulence and diabetes-related morbidities in subjects. Different key metabolic organs and pathways have been surveyed to comprehend the basic components of these impacts. Beneath, we have illustrated the effect of IF on metabolically significant organs, of which their improved capacity may present foundational medical advantages in mouse models.

Fat tissue is a key metabolic organ; in this manner understanding its reaction to IF is critical to uncover the instruments of IF-intervened metabolic advantages. Notwithstanding fat-mass decrease, numerous examinations in subject have shown that IF advances sound changes in the fat tissue. An investigation exhibited that CR in subject brings about expanded articulation of qualities related with the thermogenic capacity of earthy colored fat (e.g., uncoupling protein-1, a key thermogenic quality, in the future Ucp1) inside the white fat tissue (WAT), which was initiated through expanded kind 2 invulnerable reaction and Sirt1 articulation. Not long after, two autonomous examinations showed that 2:1 isocaloric and 1:1 IF instigates WAT searing through actuation of mitigating macrophage polarization and acceptance of miniature biome-created metabolites, individually. Essentially, isocaloric two times every day-taking care of routine likewise advanced WAT searing, upgraded mitochondrial biogenesis, and expanded WAT oxygen utilization rate, surveyed by tissue respirometry. These investigations propose that the caloric sum, yet regulation of the eating design itself changes entire body digestion through acceptance of WAT thermogenesis and decrease in adiposity. Also, IF up manages CDC-like kinase 2 (CLK2) in earthy colored fat tissue (BAT) in postprandial conditions to invigorate Ucp1 articulation, consequently improving eating regimen instigated thermogenesis (38).

Last, IF was demonstrated to be related with tweaks in different adipokines, remembering increments for adiponectin and neuregulin 4 (Nrg4), and decreases in leptin and resistin, which may all be related with metabolic upgrades in different tissues. In hereditarily fat subject (ob/ob, leptin-inadequate subject), an investigation has exhibited that 60% CR prompted diminished body weight, improved fat thermogenesis, and upgraded insulin affectability. In any case, a new report showed that 19 days of ADF (comprising of 37% CR) didn't bring about altogether diminished body weight in ob/ob creatures, notwithstanding enhancements in glucose homeostasis and improved insulin affectability. Additionally, multi week of isocaloric IF in ob/ob subject was not compelling in decreasing body weight, and IF-oppressed ob/ob creatures neglected to actuate beiging or show changes in fat resistant profile. Be that as it may, these creatures displayed upgraded postprandial insulin discharge, which was joined by expanded plasma GLP-1 levels. This proposes that a more thorough caloric limitation might be needed for the advantageous impacts of IF in instances of extreme weight.

As a critical organ in processing and assimilation of supplements, diet profoundly affects intestinal recovery and ancestor cell work. An investigation has shown that a solitary 24-hours quick expands intestinal immature microorganism work, demonstrated by upgraded organoid-framing limit, by driving a powerful PPAR-intervened unsaturated fat oxidation program. This recommends that drawn out dietary mediations could fundamentally improve intestinal immature microorganism capacity and digestion. To be sure, CR expanded Olfm 4 crude intestinal begetters just as Paneth cells by actuating mTORC1 and Sirt1 in Paneth cells. Additionally, it was shown that intestinal miniature biota displays diurnal motions, which are impacted by taking care of rhythms, and interruption in this rhythmicity is related with metabolic aggravations (88). Accordingly adjustments in gut miniature biome by dietary mediation might be essential since they are straightforwardly connected with improved metabolic homeostasis. To be sure, ADF considerably adjusted gut miniature biome arrangement, with huge enlistment of miniature biome-created acetic acid derivation and lactate metabolites. Besides, transplantation of IF-oppressed miniature biota was adequate to improve stoutness related metabolic dysfunctions. Besides, IF improved indications of a various sclerosis model by upgrading gut microbial variety and modifying their metabolic pathways, including sugar and lipid digestion. The creators have shown that IF expanded gut administrative T cells and diminished IL-17-delivering T cells, which was related with decreased fiery cytokine levels in fringe blood. Essentially, FMD decreased foundational and intestinal irritation, expanded Lgr 5 intestinal immature microorganism number, and invigorated the bounty of defensive gut microbial families. Significantly, FMD turned around DSS-initiated intestinal pathogenesis, and fecal transfer from FMD-treated subject was discovered to be adequate in relieving side effects of provocative gut infection (IBD).

In clinical settings, IF and CR mediations are principally proceeded as helpful systems to diminish body weight and improve metabolic boundaries in hefty as well as diabetic people. Albeit unique IF regimens have been clinically tried, ADF stays to be the most-examined intercession. Numerous investigations reliably show advantages of present moment (8–multi week) ADF in stout people, remembering decrease for body weight and fat mass, and diminishes in fatty substances and aggregate and LDL cholesterol. Nonetheless, ADF has effect HDL cholesterol levels. Also, a 5:2 IF concentrate in fat female people announced decreases in body weight, fasting insulin, and homeostasis model evaluation of insulin opposition (HOMA-IR) following 3 and a half year.

Preliminaries in non-large or somewhat overweight people showed comparative outcomes following a month of ADF with decreases in body weight, fat mass, cardiovascular danger, and enlistment of beta-hydroxybutyrate (characteristic of ketosis). This proposes that, even in sound people, IF could fill in as a defensive system to keep up solid body weight and generally speaking metabolic wellbeing.

Despite the fact that TRF preliminaries have announced comparative advantages to ADF, body-weight reduction was not seen in all examinations, proposing that a more tough dietary limitation might be needed to notice decreases in body weight. In spite of the shortfall of weight reduction, glucose homeostasis was improved in a few examinations, and one investigation announced a decrease in a variety of provocative markers in plasma (e.g., IL-1, IL-6, and IGF-1). This recommends that, despite the fact that IF regimens that include CR might be more proficient in decreasing body weight, basically changing eating example to join a more extended fasting period might be adequate to improve metabolic boundaries even without generally speaking caloric admission decrease.

Albeit fat tissue thermogenesis has been featured as a driving system of IF-interceded metabolic upgrades, its progressions in people because of dietary mediations are to a great extent obscure. An 8-week CR mediation was appeared to decrease body weight and fat mass in overweight ladies and men yet didn't incite cooking in subcutaneous WAT. Furthermore, changes in muscle versus fat and insulin obstruction were free of changes in WAT cooking markers. Maybe, they showed sex and occasional varieties in earthy colored and beige fat markers in human subcutaneous WAT. This inconsistency might be generally established in the degree of command over ecological conditions. Despite the fact that food admission and lodging climate (temperature and circadian rhythms) are firmly controlled in mouse examines, these are profoundly variation in clinical examination. Especially, temperature significantly affects cooking of WAT under IF intercession. A new report showed that subject exposed to thermo nonpartisan condition (30°C) preferred addresses human energy digestion over those at encompassing temperature (20 to 22°C). Surely, subject exposed to IF in thermo nonpartisan condition actually showed decreased body weight and improved glucose homeostasis without searing of WAT, emulating the metabolic impacts saw in human IF considers. Accordingly building up ideal conditions for IF would be a fundamental advance toward adjusting creature studies to clinical examination. By and by, both mouse and human's examinations present positive metabolic impacts upon IF.

Cardiovascular infection (CVD) is at present the main source of death all around the world. Control of modifiable danger factors like smoking, active work, weight, and helpless dietary propensities can improve cardiovascular wellbeing and diminishing the worldwide predominance of CVD.

Creature models have recently shown decreases in resting pulse and circulatory strain in light of IF. An investigation announced that IF improves cardiovascular transformation to push, with weakened circulatory strain (BP) and pulse because of outside stressors and a more quick recuperation to standard levels. Unthinkingly, CR and IF diminish oxidative pressure in the myocardium, with diminished oxidative changes of proteins and DNA, just as diminished lipid peroxidation. Furthermore, IF diminished provocative reaction and the quantity of apoptotic myocytes in a myocardial localized necrosis (MI) model, with lessened post-MI heart rebuilding. Besides, IF was appeared to improve plasma lipid profile by lessening LDL cholesterol. Subsequently IF may improve cardiovascular wellbeing by tweaking pulse, circulatory strain, and lipid digestion in creature models.

In people, there is an overall agreement that IF improves cardiovascular wellbeing because of enhancements in plasma lipid and provocative marker profile. As referenced over, a few clinical investigations have shown that ADF lessens plasma triacylglycerol, aggregate and LDL cholesterol level, with intermittentities in HDL level change. By and large, discoveries uncover that improved plasma lipid profile might be intelligent of cardio defensive impacts of IF in people. Besides, high BP is a regular measure and determinant of CVD hazard. Eight to twelve weeks of ADF in stout people prompted diminished systolic BP or decreased systolic and diastolic BP. A drawn out investigation likewise showed that 5:2 IF for a half year prompted diminishes in both systolic and diastolic BP). As of late, a directed controlled taking care of clinical preliminary utilized isocaloric early

TRF (6-hours taking care of window, with last dinner before 3 PM) for multi week in pre-diabetic men. After the 5-week intercession, the resting pulse, systolic and diastolic BP, complete cholesterol level, and serum oxidative pressure markers were definitely brought down. Comparative outcomes were acquired in a clinical preliminary utilizing 1 day/week fasting IF routine in non-fat and stout ladies, where 3 multi week of IF prompted diminished absolute cholesterol, LDL cholesterol, and TG levels, however not changes in BP. These differing brings about cardiovascular boundaries might be credited to the force and span of intercessions, the cardio metabolic conditions, and the hereditary foundation of members. In general, IF diminishes the danger of CVD with upgrades in plasma lipid profile, and decrease in pulse and BP in the two subjects and people.

Invulnerable framework brokenness is at the focal point of maturing and a scope of threatening sicknesses including disease. Since dietary intercessions significantly affect entire body digestion, including immunometabolism, IF-interceded modifications in the safe framework may give understanding into its helpful efficacies for malignancy treatment and avoidance.

In subjects, drawn out fasting (PF; fasting more than 48–120 hour) has been appeared to upgrade hematopoietic recovery, as shown by expanded protection of hematopoietic foundational microorganisms and improved recuperation from chemotherapy-initiated decrease of lymphoid cells. PF has shown a decrease in circling insulin-like development factor 1 (IGF-1), a key cytokine associated with the underlying development and upkeep of tumors. Intermittent CR decreased mammary tumor occurrence and postponed tumor movement in the MMTV-TGF bosom malignant growth model, which was related with diminished serum leptin levels. Also, TRF in MMTV-PYMT bosom disease model exposed to HFD stifled tumor development and decreased plasma convergences of key markers, for example, leptin. TRF (dull stage confined taking care of) was appeared to lessen weight initiated metastasis of Lewis lung carcinoma, in which the essential tumor showed its own circadian rhythmicity and straightforwardly reacted to eating-design adjustments. A potential clarification for IF-interceded tumor development delay is that fasting incites enactment of SIRT3, which directs receptive oxygen species (ROS) levels and eventually blunts the NLRP3 inflammasome pathway. Since the inflammasome is a critical component in intrinsic insusceptible actuation and tissue irritation, impeding its initiation may assume a part in lessening introductory disease development. Like PF, numerous creature considers have likewise shown that CR and FMD lessen circling IGF-1 levels. Interestingly, it has been accounted for that intermittent CR changed tumor energy digestion from oxidative phosphorylation to glycolysis, bringing about expanded flowing disease immature microorganisms and procurement of epithelial-mesenchymal progress aggregate during the post-starvation time frame. This recommends that post-starvation food overconsumption can rather upgrade tumor development and might be related with threatening metastasis. In synopsis, the part of IF in tumor beginning movement actually stays dubious; in this manner, future examination is justified to test the effect of IF on tumorigenesis.

In people, weight is related with expanded danger of different malignant growth types, including bosom, pancreatic, liver, and prostate disease. A decrease in body weight by means of dietary intercessions, for example, IF may lessen the pervasiveness and movement of malignancy. In any case, until now, there are no human investigations straightforwardly connecting the effect of IF to malignancy. One examination researched fasting-related disease clinical results by exposing patients to pre-oral carb load or a 24-hours quick before bosom malignancy medical procedure. Abstained ER-positive patients displayed improved repeat free endurance and clinical result in 88 months of follow-up. To comprehend the component, we audit the impacts of IF on different disease hazard biomarkers that add to the etiology and advancement of malignancy. For example, higher muscle to fat ratio mass is related with expanded danger of obtrusive bosom malignancy in post-menopausal ladies. Delayed evening time fasting was demonstrated to be related with improved glycemic control and diminished malignant growth biomarkers, giving a basic and non-pharmacological technique for lessening the danger of bosom disease pervasiveness and repeat. Different malignancy biomarkers, for example, plasma adipokines and provocative cytokines are likewise affected by IF. For instance, TRF and ADF have appeared to fundamentally expand plasma adiponectin level, which has been related with diminished pervasiveness of prostate malignant growth, colorectal disease, endometrial malignancy, and bosom disease. Curiously, adiponectin level is contrarily associated with a few incendiary cytokines, for example, IL-

6, TNF, and IFN. Since persistent aggravation fills in as a central member in the improvement of malignant growth, expanded calming adiponectin instigated by IF may advance an enemy of tumor microenvironment. Frequently expanded by heftiness, the adipokine leptin was accounted for to have a supportive of provocative job and is related with more elevated levels of fiery cytokines, more prominent neutrophil initiation, and expanded ROS level. Dietary regimens of ADF and 6:1 IF (1 day of fasting each week) decreased circling leptin levels, and 2:1 IF essentially diminished Lep articulation in the fat tissue. All in all, tweak of different adipokines by IF may give mitigating tissue microenvironment that may forestall the improvement of different tumors.

Weight reduction with IF and CR diminishes coursing levels of C-responsive protein, which is a sign of aggravation. Likewise, a few examinations detailed that Ramadan fasting, a particular strict fasting routine, prompted decreased degrees of IL-1, IL-6, and TNF. In sound volunteers, fasting prompted less NLRP3 inflammasome enactment, as demonstrated by diminished discharge of IL-1, IL-18, and TNF from essential monocytes disengaged from abstained subjects, and re-taking care of switched this aggregate. Nonetheless, numerous examinations have in any case announced that IF regimens had no impact on flowing incendiary cytokines. Together, these investigations exhibit intermittentities in provocative boundaries, which brings up issues in regards to the precision of techniques for distinguishing circling cytokine levels and the ramifications of changes in these boundaries in general metabolic wellbeing.

3.5 Intermittent Fasting Effects on the Nervous System

A few advantageous impacts of dietary limitation regimens on neurobehavioral capacities in subjects have been archived. For instance, age-related decrease in execution in a labyrinth task and locomotor movement was forestalled by CR. Other mouse examines have additionally announced better engine and memory execution at 15 and 22 months old enough. Whenever improved engine coordination and intellectual capacity in maturing subjects through upgraded mitochondrial action and diminished oxidative harm in the cerebrum. Upon openness to neurotoxin, IF-oppressed subjects showed expanded opposition of neurons in the hippocampus, recommending improved safeguarding of neural cells within the sight of exogenous stressors. Likewise, CR expanded endurance of recently produced neurons from hippocampus undeveloped cells, which improved synaptic versatility and generally speaking cerebrum work. In hereditary models of Alzheimer's illness, creatures exposed to CR or IF displayed upgraded exploratory conduct and better execution in securing and maintenance assignments. Specifically, the CR bunch showed diminished aggregation of beta-amyloid peptide and phospho-tau articulation, which are signs of neuropathology. All the more as of late, an examination has shown that IF enhances clinical pathology of numerous sclerosis model by miniature biome-intervened decrease in focal sensory system (CNS) irritation and demyelination. The advantageous impact of IF in different neurodegenerative illnesses might be ascribed to expanded degree of neuroprotective cytokines, for example, mind determined neurotropic factor (BDNF), which is related with decreased ischemic cerebrum harm and improvement of by and large mind wellbeing. In hereditarily stout/diabetic db/db subject (leptin receptor-lacking subject), IF had the option to forestall diabetic intricacies, for example, diabetic retinopathy by expanding neuroprotective bile corrosive digestion through changes in the gut miniature biome, which focuses on the ganglion cell layer and secures against retinal degeneration. Moreover, a new report has shown that

SIRT3 is significant in versatile upgrade of GABAergic synaptic transmission for transformation to IF, recommending the immediate effect of dietary changes in the CNS capacity and wellbeing.

Decrease of intellectual capacity has been related with corpulence. Ongoing examinations have shown that absence of activity joined with helpless dietary practices are hazard factors for neurodegenerative sicknesses like Alzheimer's illness. Also, IF decidedly impacts on neurocognitive capacity in subjects. Despite the fact that there are no human examinations tending to the immediate impacts of IF on the sensory system, there are contemplates that recommend the possible positive effect of dietary mediations on neurocognitive capacity in people. In an investigation, typical or overweight old people were exposed to 3 months of a 30% CR. Following their intercession, the members showed critical improvement in verbal memory contrasted and the control partner. In any case, level of BDNF, regularly connected with diminished neural brokenness and degeneration, stayed unaltered. In spite of the fact that BDNF levels were frequently expanded in subjects following dietary intercessions, this factor is hard to precisely evaluate in a clinical setting, since serum levels may not be demonstrative of levels inside the mind. To see whether the advantages of fasting intercessions for Alzheimer's sicknesses are clinically translatable, a human eating regimen mediation study has started a stage 1 clinical preliminary, where Alzheimer's patients will go through FMD, and variety of IF, to survey its viability as a therapy.

Albeit the impacts of IF are all the more completely investigated in preclinical examinations, clinical exploration additionally has shown advantages of dietary changes on improving psychological capacity, justifying further investigation into the remedial capability of dietary mediations.

3.6 Discussion and Future Directions

Despite the fact that IF as a methods for weight the board and upgrades in entire body digestion is acquiring notoriety, fasting for social and strict intentions has been polished for a long time. For instance, the Ramadan quick is a particular type of strict IF rehearsed by a large number of Muslims in Islamic culture. During the long stretch of Ramadan, Muslims avoid all types of caloric admission for 12–14 hours among dawn and dusk consistently for a 29-to 30-day time frame. Subsequently the Ramadan quick gives a fantastic chance to investigate the impacts of IF in an enormous populace. Studies have shown diminishes in body weight and coursing supportive of provocative cytokines during Ramadan. Conversely, there are examines showing negligible medical advantages and restricted maintainability of Ramadan fasting, specifically in solid people. This conflicting finding of fasting during Ramadan might be credited to upset circadian musicality. Fasting during the day (dynamic stage) and eating in the evening (latent stage) negates chemical discharge, rest, and actual coordination designs related with the circadian rhythmicity. These perceptions demonstrate that the circadian planning of eating/fasting would be vital to streamline IF routine just as to decide the adequacy of IF.

In the event that mediations in subjects have reliably shown helpful impacts, for example, weight reduction, expanded insulin affectability, and improved metabolic and cardiovascular profile. Notwithstanding the shocking number of preclinical models exhibiting these positive effects, clinical examinations still can't seem to reliably imitate these outcomes. This inconsistency between preclinical models and human preliminaries might be ascribed to a misfortune in severe ecological control from a research facility to a clinical setting. Puzzling components like hereditary inclination, over a significant time span metabolic status, age, sex, amount of energy admission, and warm climate may likewise impact clinical preliminary outcomes. Moreover, contrasted and preclinical models, where IF reads keep going for quite a long time, human IF reads are performed for a moderately transient time of 4 multi week. This may clarify the intermittentities in clinical results and generally peripheral upgrades, as a more thorough and long haul dietary intercession might be needed to notice clinically critical enhancements. All the more significantly, quantitative measures got from complete phenotyping, and broad tissue and plasma profiling of preclinical models are missing in human preliminaries and in this manner neglect to show fundamental and tissue-explicit physiological impacts of IF in people. Such quantitative measures are restricted to fundamental metabolic boundaries and serum investigation because of the idea of clinical examinations, accordingly possibly recommending physiological ramifications on IF intercessions in people, which may not precisely mirror the impacts of IF.

Despite the fact that IF has substantiated itself as a promising intercession in preclinical models, further examination is needed to depict the expected advantages in a clinical setting. To assess its remedial viability for people, thorough controls should be carried out to represent differing components like quality and amount of energy consumption, warm climate, hereditary cosmetics, rest examples, current and earlier metabolic status, achievability, and manageability. Controlling these target gauges and expanding test size should help reveal the clinically ideal length of IF, just as expected unfriendly impacts, like hypoglycemia, passionate crabbiness, body weight recapture following end of IF routine. With additional examination into its viability among people, IF can possibly be an amazingly open and appealing restorative intercession for people expecting to improve their metabolic, intellectual, and cardiovascular wellbeing through nonsurgical and non-pharmacological methodologies.

Conclusion

For fasting to be in excess of a weight reduction craze, more prominent logical thoroughness is required from interventional preliminaries than is found in the writing. While energy for fasting is expanding, clinical significance stays low on account of inadequate human information, including practically nonexistent controlled preliminaries, not many clinical results examines, absence of adjustment for swelled sort I blunder rates from various speculation tests, and restricted security information. The proof recommends, in any case, that restorative fasting may give generous advantage to diminishing clinical danger.

Lightning Source UK Ltd.
Milton Keynes UK
UKHW022004030621
384904UK00002B/404

9 781802 265507